The Art of
Living
Well
with
Crohn's

Bardolf & Company

The Art of Living Well with Crohn's

ISBN 978-1-938842-12-2
Copyright © 2013 by John T. Johns

Published by Bardolf & Company
5430 Colewood Pl.
Sarasota, FL 34232
941-232-0113
www.bardolfandcompany.com

Cover design by Shaw Creative
www.shawcreativegroup.com

Cover photo of author by Colette Johns

The Art of
Living
Well
with
Crohn's

John T. Johns

Bardolf & Company
Sarasota, Florida

❧ TABLE OF CONTENTS

**To Colette
my wife
and best friend**

The art of living lies less in eliminating
our troubles than in growing with them.

—Bernard M. Baruch

✣ PREFACE

In 1979, Dr. Hay, a radiologist with about 40 years of experience under his belt, told me I had Crohn's disease. He looked very concerned and said he was sorry. I had never had a personal connection with the word "disease" before, but that day, I felt like I had been hit by a Mike Tyson sucker punch. I had an illness, a chronic disease that wouldn't go away.

Crohn's disease is an inflammatory bowel disease, also called regional enteritis, meaning inflammation of the intestines. In the past, it has been described as an autoimmune disorder, but is now considered an immune deficiency, in which the immune system attacks healthy tissue.

Dr. Hay mentioned that it also was called "Ike's disease" because our 34th president, Dwight D. Eisenhower, had the disease. Immediately, my mind raced through what I knew about him. He served two terms as President of the United States. He was a famous general, commanding the Allied forces during WWII. He liked to play golf. He had several heart attacks, dying of the last one at age 78.

I said, "Well, he lived a good life!"

The doctor's look of concern lightened up, and with a trace of a smile, he said, "Yes, I believe he did."

Fast forward 34 years. By now, I had lived more than half of my life with Crohn's disease. I sat in the office of my gastroenterologist, who had been helping me deal with a flare-up, my first in over 7 years. He looked at me and said, "Your lab tests look great. You know, you really are a very healthy guy."

Not long after, I took a stress test. There were five of us altogether, and the young cardiologist monitored us on separate computer screens. She began to focus on me, asking me questions about running and exercise. Her comment to the room was, "I want to be like him when I grow up."

I have spent some time thinking about what these two doctors had said and about the neighbors, young and old, that consider me and my wife the active ones in our community. I sail, I run, I go camping, I have an active social life and so much more. True, being diagnosed with Crohn's disease means my life has changed fundamentally. Things that I took for granted, such as eating an apple, required modification. My close relationships have been affected positively and negatively. They certainly did not stay the same. Even casual relationships haven't been immune to change. Although I can't say I'm on friendly terms with my Crohn's disease, I accept it as a part of my day-to-day existence. More importantly, I refuse to let it run my life.

The purpose of this book is to give everyone who has Crohn's information about how to live with and manage the disease for the best life possible. While I have included a lot of personal stories, it is more than an anecdotal account. Almost everything that I have used in my struggle with Crohn's is backed up with scientific studies.

My doctors have told me that most of their patients do not want to change their behavior regarding their disease, but if you are someone that believes you can make a difference in your life if given half a chance, this book is for you. They also tell me that what works for one will not necessarily work for another. I quote from studies so that the reader will know that a certain behavior is working for many, not just for me or a few unique cases.

A number of individuals that deal with chronic health problems have told me that they have met too many people who claim to have all the answers, along with an evangelical attitude, and that can be annoying. At the same time, they have found that there are so many of "the answers" that they do not know who or what to believe. That's why I have tried to keep things simple and straight forward, rather than overwhelm with a flood of detailed information.

What qualifies a layman like me to write a book about managing Crohn's disease? Simply this: even though I have had serious problems with Crohn's, through my own studies, and trial and error, I have learned to cope with it quite well. The problems have gradually become less the longer I have it and I have been able to live a great life.

This book is not about trying to save or cure you. It does not contain a silver lining. It is not about a pill, a medical procedure, a supplement, or any single behavioral change that will solve all Crohn's problems. Instead, it is about lifestyle adjustments that are easy to do on a regular basis, if you make the effort. I want to give you information backed up by experience and scientific data that will allow you to manage your Crohn's disease, just as I have.

I now have many different means of coping. Some, I first tried because I believed they would help. Others, I was already doing or started for reasons that had nothing to do with Crohn's, and only later did I learn or realize how important they were to my management of the disease. I have always been a physically active person, so exercising is almost part of my nature. I explored yoga because I thought it would be good for me, but had no idea how helpful it would become in dealing with Crohn's. Changes in diet and stress management activities became part of my arsenal as a result of research.

This book explains what the choices are, how they benefit someone with Crohn's, how they benefited me, and the coping skills I have learned from a lifetime of working with them. It also explains, in layman terms, some of the scientific basis for why they are important for someone dealing with a chronic health issue or with Crohn's specifically. When the research is not Crohn's specific, I use my own experience and rationale for why it is useful for those of us who are challenged with Crohn's disease in particular. I also give information on how to implement these behaviors and/or give sources for guidance or instruction when it is not practical in a book of this nature to go into that much detail.

From one Chronie to another, I want your life to be as good and as exciting as mine has been.

🌿 *Chapter 1*
MY STORY

*Person with one health problem is often more
healthy than person with no health problem.*
—Chinese Proverb

I was 33 when I was diagnosed with Crohn's disease. I was living in Murfreesboro, Tennessee, at the time and my life was packed full. I had recently completed an MBA on the GI Bill, having served 3 years in the army, including a one-year tour in Vietnam as a first lieutenant. I bought a house, got married, and went through the process of getting legal custody of my sons in another state. I ran a janitorial service that I had started while in grad school, and tried to figure out my career path. I also liked to play tennis once or twice a week in the spring, summer and fall, and racquetball in the off season. My philosophy was simple: work hard, play hard.

One day in 1978, I decided to stop at a medical clinic to get something for my hemorrhoids. They had never been a problem before, but I had been having a lot of diarrhea lately. I didn't consider it a big deal, certainly not important enough to see my regular doctor. The clinic was convenient, perfect for a busy man like me.

When they put me on the scales, I was surprised, no, in disbelief, to see I weighed only 133 pounds. At just under 6 feet tall, I had weighed around 165 pounds since I was a senior in high school. The doctor on call checked me out and decided I needed some valium. I knew something was wrong with me, but I was pretty sure it wasn't my nerves.

I never filled that prescription, but I made an appointment with my regular doctor, an internal medicine physician. The in-office procedure, a rigid sigmoidoscopy exam, showed nothing, so he sent me for a series of GI tract tests. I was X-rayed from the mouth down to my toes, including a barium enema. The latter led to the diagnosis of Crohn's disease. My doctor prescribed Azulfidine, a combination of sulfur and aspirin, and according to him, the drug of choice at the time. In fact, Azulfidine became my maintenance treatment until 2004. From time to time when I had an acute flare-up, I often used Prednisone, a synthetic steroid that acts as an immune suppressant.

The first few years following my diagnosis were a roller coaster. There were times when I felt so bad I thought my life as I knew it was over. I imagined what my existence would be like as an invalid, confined in a bed or a wheelchair. I figured I could always play computer chess, a game I liked, and would be able to study further. But the thought of being a burden to my wife and children was difficult to swallow. I had never thought of myself as being an overly proud man, but I had my limits. Fortunately, more often than not, everything was under control. True, my health was not perfect but the medicines were working. I could play some tennis, work hard, and take care of my family. Life, for the most part, was pretty good.

By then, 7 years after my initial diagnosis, I was engaged in a new career. I owned a landscaping company with several employees. We designed, installed and maintained lawns, shrubs, trees and irrigation systems. I had several employees. I'm the kind of person who loves to do a lot of different things. I spent about half my time on the administrative side, designing, bookkeeping, processing payroll, creating sales, maintaining accounts payable, etc. The other half, I worked on the job, making sure it was done efficiently and professionally. I was a hands-on manager and would do the physical labor if I was caught up on my other responsibilities or we needed more labor to get the job done. Like most entrepreneurs, I put in many more than 40 hours a week.

One Friday morning, it started to rain and rain hard, which meant no outside work. The employees loved a Friday off. I did too, so I handed out checks and shut down shop for the rest of the week. I was hungry and stopped on the way home at one of the burger chain restaurants. I ordered a double burger with cheese and bacon, a Coke and French fries. Boy, it was good.

At home, sated and enjoying the sound of the rain, I soon fell asleep on the couch. An hour or two later, I got up to go to the bathroom. Crash! I passed out and fell. When I came to and tried to get up—crash!—I went down again. After the fourth time, I decided to call someone to take me to the hospital. When my ride pulled up, I literally crawled out to the car. Initially, I was okay as long as I didn't stand up.

It turned out that I was dehydrated because of a blockage in my intestines. Blood is in short supply when the body is dehydrated. The brain, to protect itself and get the blood supply it needs, forces one to pass out. Falling and being on the ground allows more blood to get to the brain and if the head didn't hit anything on the way down, the brain remains unharmed and back in business. Ingenious, but annoying! Luckily, I suffered no real damage.

At the only city hospital, I learned that my regular doctor was out of town on vacation and that Dr. X was taking care of his patients. Dr. X was not the most respected doctor around, but I didn't know that at the time. After a couple of days of suffering with forced throwing up, where the vomit is projected across the room, another doctor convinced Dr. X to order a tube put through my nose and throat and into my stomach and to put me on steroids. The steroids sounded fine, but a tube down my throat was pretty scary. I managed it after gagging a few times, and it wasn't so bad until a couple of days later when my throat got really sore. Eventually, I was on my way home and back to work.

But 2 months later, I was back in the hospital after passing out again. Even though I swore to myself I would never use Dr. X again,

I saw him in the hall and being in considerable pain, asked him to come into the examining room. This time I was able to accept the tube going down the throat without gagging. It wasn't even that bad going down. Ironically, just before I had called the doctor in, my wife had been telling the hospital staff we would see any doctor except Dr. X. He had overheard her and, either because of his pride or his desire to do damage control for his reputation, I received the best care ever. In a few days, I was okay and back to work.

About a month later, I was passing out again. I dialed for help. By then, I had hit rock bottom, psychologically. I couldn't talk without sobbing. On the way to the hospital, I wept without tears. I was sure I was going to be an invalid.

My regular doctor was finally back in town and called in a new GI tract specialist, Murfreesboro's first gastroenterologist. For me, he was a ray of hope. I assumed he would have lots of specialized knowledge and skill as well as great advice. Maybe I wouldn't end up an invalid after all. But he wasn't all that different in his approach. He relied on drugs and just like my doctors during previous flair-ups, told me to eat and do whatever I wanted. However, this time I backed off a bit on his advice.

By then, I had come to understand that I had to take more responsibility for my health on my own. I realized that this bright young specialist did not have any magic pills and, while extremely helpful, had neither the time nor the knowledge to make me healthy enough to live a decent life. I had three not very pleasant stays in the hospital in just a few months, and I was determined it wasn't going to continue that way. I didn't yet understand the extent of the power I had in fighting Crohn's disease. I vowed to be more engaged in the battles and eventually understood that my actions and decisions were as important as my doctor's.

I began seeing the gastroenterologist monthly for vitamin B-12 shots and general checkups. He would listen to my gut. If my bowel sounds were weak, indicating constriction, he ordered X-rays to be taken and often prescribed Prednisone, as well as weekly visits, until the gut opened up. Lucky for me, he always got me off the steroids as soon as possible.

A graduate from the highly-respected Vanderbilt Medical School, he had just completed his residency and was well up to date on the latest Crohn's treatment. Confident and driven, he thought medicine was the only answer to my problems. He didn't believe that diet had any effect on Crohn's disease. Figuring that stress was a normal part of life, he never mentioned I might consider learning how to manage it.

So, now I had a specialist I liked and respected. There was just one catch; I was still on the same track. I never traveled out of town without some Prednisone in my pocket. I still worked and played hard, but I backed off a little and was a little more careful about what I ate.

Three years later I had to have emergency surgery. Three and a half feet of my small intestine, including my ileum, were removed. I was taken off all medications. I understood that Crohn's almost always returns after surgery. I had even read that if it doesn't come back, it wasn't really Crohn's disease. Therefore, I was disappointed, but not surprised when a few weeks later, the diagnosis came back positive. I was put back on Azulfidine.

I was 43 years old and figured I was on track to have surgery every 10 years or so. I joked that if I lost 3 ½ feet each time, I could make it to age 100 before I ran out of small intestine. Still, it didn't sound all that great, so I decided to try a new approach. First, I gradually began to change my diet. I started going to Wendy's instead of McDonald's and Burger King because I could get baked potatoes instead of French fries and the hamburgers were not as greasy. I started observing what I ate and how it affected me. I tried to cut back on greasy food and red meat, eating more chicken. Years later, I decided to do without meat altogether and become a vegetarian. (I shed more light on my dietary research in Chapter 4.)

Changing my lifestyle was a subtle process that took place over a period of several years. I ate a healthier diet and started practicing yoga at home, doing a 15 to 30 minute routine before work.

Before my surgery, I had been attending a weekly yoga class, not because of the philosophical or spiritual aspects, but because I believed my athletic pursuits would be better served if I stretched more. While playing racquetball a few years earlier, I had ruptured my Achilles tendon. The surgical repair had been successful, but I knew I needed to stretch my entire body as well as the repaired tendon. Yoga proved to be much more than a means of increasing my range of motion. Eventually, it became a big part of my Crohn's management.

Just before I turned 50, my life took another big turn. My sixteen-year marriage was coming to an end. The landscaping business was doing great, but it didn't provide much satisfaction anymore. I think I thrive on challenges, and although I enjoyed the success, I found the routine stifling. So I sold the business and began the process of developing a new career.

I went to San Francisco, studied yoga for 2 years and became a certified instructor. When I returned to Tennessee, I opened a yoga studio and started to hold classes. Later, I completed a 600-hour course in Tennessee and became a licensed therapeutic massage therapist as well. I wanted to learn all I could about the body and how to make it healthy.

The effect of yoga on my overall health, not just on my Crohn's disease, was dramatic. My posture greatly improved. Even my bowed legs were less bowed. There is no doubt in my mind that the process of opening up my body with yoga got rid of toxins that were stored there. The process of doing yoga also encourages the mind to be more open to new ideas. The more I studied yoga, the healthier my lifestyle became, especially as it related to diet and stress.

A couple of years after opening my yoga studio, I met Colette, who became my wife. She was a massage therapist, an organic gardener, a great cook and a vegetarian. Not only did she love camping and the outdoors, she had a spirit of adventure. Years earlier, she had overcome some serious health challenges of her own and, like me, had to live a healthy lifestyle. She found the book, *Eating Right for a Bad Gut*, by Dr. James Scala. It took two readings for its wisdom and knowledge to fully penetrate. Since then it has helped bring my Crohn's management to another level.

In 2005, Colette and I moved to Southwest Florida. I cut back on yoga but increased my time spent in nature and doing aerobic exercise. Taking fish oils, eating a very healthy diet, and living a healthy lifestyle allowed me to get off of medications.

But then, I got careless. True to my impulsive nature, I thought I could be less mindful and do just as well. Over the next 7 years, I gave up my disciplined, moderate lifestyle. It was a downward spiral that resulted in ever more frequent days when I felt fatigued and unable to do much. I had annual physicals and an excellent general practitioner as my doctor, but I realized that maybe it was time again for a gut specialist.

In June of 2011, I met with a new gastroenterologist. My energy level had been quite low for a couple of months. In retrospect, it had been more off than on for almost a whole year. The doctor prescribed Asacol and told me to come back in 2 weeks, if I was still having problems. At that point, he would probably prescribe my old stand-by, Prednisone.

When I went to see him 2 weeks later, I was amazed and annoyed to learn he was on vacation. Upset, but proactive, I went to my regular doctor and he wrote a prescription for Prednisone. On the recommendation of one of my wife's friends, I scheduled an appointment with another gastroenterologist. He was great. The first office visit with him lasted 30 minutes, unusual in Florida, where the average time spent with a doctor is less than 7 minutes! After a colonoscopy, digestive tract X-rays, and a couple of rounds of steroids, we settled on Asacol for my maintenance medication. He and his assistant got me back on track, and I've been in good shape ever since.

So the question is, has Crohn's been a gift or a curse in my life? The disease has placed some limits on what I do and what I eat, and it has robbed me of considerable energy. At the same time, it has provided me with many gifts, including humility, greater flexibility in facing daily challenges, and satisfaction in achievements with a "handicap." I think in many ways I am healthier for it because I had to be more health conscious.

I have become a practitioner of moderation. I run a little, bicycle a bit, do some sailing and camping, engage in socializing, occasionally drink beer or wine, and eat great tasting foods. I practice yoga and meditation. Colette and I limit eating out, not only because it is expensive, but because I often pay the price later on in other ways. Yes, I have had Crohn's disease for 35 years, and I have to be prudent in what I do, but I live a great life; and I believe many others with Crohn's can do so, too.

Chapter 2
CROHN'S DISEASE BASICS

As an inflammatory disease that attacks the digestive tract, Crohn's can occur anywhere from the mouth to the bowels. Most cases involve the ileum (last section of the small intestine), the colon (large intestine) or the upper small intestine and stomach. Symptoms may include abdominal pain, diarrhea, vomiting and weight loss, as well as skin rashes and arthritis.

The disease is named after Dr. Burrill B. Crohn, a New York City gastroenterologist who published an important paper with two colleagues in 1932, describing what was then a relatively little known condition. It could have been named after others who did work on it earlier, but Crohn's is the name that stuck.

More than 700,000 Americans suffer from the disease, which strikes both genders equally. The peak period of its onset is ages 15 to 30. There is a relatively safe period until the fifties to seventies, but no age group is immune. I was diagnosed when I was 33 years old.

While the cause of the disease is still unknown, the fact that there are more than 30 genes associated with Crohn's suggests a strong hereditary connection. Someone who has a sibling with Crohn's has a 30 times greater chance of getting the disease than the rest of the population. But there are also environmental causes. People who smoke are twice as likely to get Crohn's as non-smokers. Living in an industrialized part of the world increases the risk of getting the disease. There is evidence that link it with diet and some medications, such as birth control pills. The stress associated with a modern lifestyle may also be a factor.

Conventional treatment for Crohn's is antibiotics and/or anti-inflammatory drugs. Because antibiotics are detrimental to the good bacteria in the intestines, doctors prescribe them sparingly and only as necessary.

The anti-inflammatory drugs primarily fall into two categories—aminosalicylates and corticosteroids. The aminosalicylates are chemically related to aspirin—the side effects are relatively mild, and most people can tolerate them for a long time. Corticosteroids like Prednisone have more serious side effects and are used only for acute flare-ups. For that reason, and because they lose their effectiveness over time, they are given for short periods of time. If medications are not effective, immune suppressing drugs may be prescribed. As a last resort, surgery may be required.

I have had all of the above and will briefly relate my experience with each, but I must caution that what works or doesn't work for one person may affect another quite differently. For that reason, working with a good physician to develop a program that suits you is essential.

Aminosalicylates

Sulfasalazine, my first medication for Crohn's, worked well for quite a few years. It is a compound made up of Sulfa, an antibiotic, and an aminosalicylic acid which is a non steroidal anti-inflammatory. I did have a fair amount of indigestion while taking the drug. I can't be certain that this was because it destroyed the good bacteria in my gut, but I always believed that to be the case. I used this medication for 26 years. After refining my diet and taking six to eight fish oil capsules per day, I was able to function well without it for almost 7 years.

When I had my flare-up in June of 2011, my doctor put me on Asacol, and I have been taking it since. I much prefer it over Sulfasalazine and have experienced no ill side effects that I am aware of. Because it does not have antibiotic qualities, my digestive tract works better. The drug is also designed to be absorbed farther down in the bowels. Because my disease is centered in the ileum, which is part of the small intestine, my doctor thought a different aminosalicylate, Pentasa, absorbed farther up, would work best for me. However, it turned out in my case that Asacol was more effective, which baffled him at first because the drug is normally prescribed for the colon rather than the small intestine.

My doctor now believes that there are one or two reasons why Asacol works for me. The valve that separates my large and small intestine was surgically removed about 10 years after my initial Crohn's diagnosis. This probably changes the pH level to make the area where my disease exists more colon like—and pH activates Asacol. Furthermore, I have a couple of ulcers in my ileum, which probably allow it to be absorbed inside the wall where my inflammation is active.

This explanation is not scientific. It is what I gathered from my doctor's comments. My experience as a patient is that prescribing medicine is sort of like a science experiment that proceeds by trial and error. You discover what works or doesn't and keep adjusting until you reach a positive conclusion. The doctors with whom I have discussed this over the years have agreed. Therefore, it is important that both doctor and patient remain flexible and not get locked into any particular drug regimen. If it works, use it; if it doesn't, try something else.

Corticosteroids

I have been taking corticosteroids—primarily Prednisone—as needed since my first Crohn's induced hospital visit. Corticosteroids do two things that can benefit a patient suffering from the disease. They reduce inflammation and suppress the immune system, preventing it from attacking certain healthy body tissue.

Side effects of corticosteroids depend on the dosage and how long they are taken. Possible side effects include glaucoma, fluid retention in the lower legs, increased blood pressure, mood swings and weight gain. Over longer periods, there is an increased possibility of developing cataracts, diabetes, and osteoporosis, as well as more infections, easier bruising and slower wound healing.

I began taking Prednisone during my first hospital visit for a blocked bowel, and off and on until my surgery 10 years later. Since then, especially after changing my diet and lifestyle, I have taken them only a handful of times. In the early years, I experienced wide mood swings—I'd get angry over things that normally I wouldn't blink an eye about. I'd have great energy at the outset and considerable fatigue when I got off the drug. Today, I don't notice those effects, but I also don't have the same dramatic positive results that I used to.

When taking corticosteroids, it is a good idea to maintain a healthy lifestyle—exercising to keep the weight gain down and to maintain strong bones and muscles, reducing calorie intake to keep off the extra weight, and taking vitamin D, and/or other supplements to reduce the risk of osteoporosis. When getting off this type of medicine, it is important to stop gradually. Tapering off will give the adrenal glands a chance to get used to the fact that they need to start producing hormones again. Quitting Prednisone too quickly may cause severe fatigue, weakness, body aches and joint pain.

Another steroid used in the treatment of Crohn's is Budesonide, which targets the terminal ileum and the right colon. It tends to have fewer side effects than Prednisone, being less damaging to bone density and having little impact on the adrenal glands. I have taken this drug once and was pleased with the results—I was able to take it for a longer period of time and didn't have to taper off as much when I stopped using it.

Vitamin B-12 Shots

My first gastroenterologist prescribed monthly shots of vitamin B-12. After some prodding, he explained that if I did not take it, serious nerve damage was possible. He said that my damaged terminal ileum may not absorb B-12, which also plays a role in preventing anemia and promotes normal growth and development. Removal of the terminal ileum is also a reason to have lifelong B-12 injections. I have been self administrating B-12 injections for about 15 years. I highly recommend learning to do this. It is not difficult and very empowering. My routine physicals include a blood test for B12 deficiency. Thankfully, I have always been in the normal range.

Immune Suppressors

Another class of drugs used in the treatment of Crohn's are the immune suppressors. I had experience with one of them, Azathioprine, in 2011 when I was dealing with a flare-up. My doctor was a big believer in this drug. I eventually decided to take it despite being concerned about some possible serious side effects, which I was told, were reversible. The doctor reminded me there were serious side effects to Crohn's, too, if it is not in remission. But when I started experiencing nausea, bloating and eventually vomiting, I took myself off the medication and called for a doctor's appointment. By the time I saw the physician assistant the next day, I was feeling better already. He put me on Prednisone, and later on, Budesonide.

My doctor thought I may have had developed pancreatitis from the Azathioprine. Had that been the case and had I stayed on it, I would have ended up in the hospital. Being proactive and discontinuing the drug saved me a lot of misery. Not waiting and insisting on an appointment with the doctor's staff ensured that things didn't get worse. Recently, a friend of mine was prescribed a sulfur drug for a non-Crohn's related infection. He ignored the warning signs and took it until he passed out and had to go to the emergency room when his throat almost closed up.

I am very glad I don't have to take one of the immune suppressors. I understand they can do great things for some people, but I don't want to take a chance with the side effects, if I don't have to.

There are other medications I have in my arsenal. Hyoscyamine, which is used to treat digestive tract ailments, works by decreasing the motion of the stomach and intestines as well as the secretion of stomach fluids, including acid. In my case, I take it as needed and have found it to be very effective when I have indigestion or bloating. When I get a little careless with my diet, a little stressed, or whatever, it is nice to have it in my medicine cabinet. I also have found that Pepto-Bismol® or baking soda sometimes work for me when Hyoscyamine will not.

Surgery

There is an old story about John Huston, the great film director who made such movies as *The Maltese Falcon*, *The Treasure of the Sierra Madre*, and *Prizzi's Honor*. When he was asked at 80 to what he attributed his longevity, he said in his crusty voice, "Surgery!"

Surgery can be an effective remedy when dealing with Crohn's disease. Personally, I have had good luck with it from the removal of my tonsils at age 4, to two hernia repairs, to the cutting out of about 3 ½ feet of my small intestines 10 years after Crohn's was diagnosed. Surgery made a huge difference in my quality of life. However, all the doctors I have known, unless they are surgeons, look at surgery as a treatment of last resort.

The primary reasons a Crohn's patient may need to go that route are an intestinal blockage, a stricture—a narrowing of the gut—extensive bleeding, a hole in the intestine, a fistula, or an abscess. In addition, surgery may be called for if a drug's side effects are intolerable or the medication is just not effective enough for an acceptable quality of life.

According to the Crohn's and Colitis Foundation of America, about two thirds to three quarters of all Crohn's patients will have surgery at some point in their lives. About one-half of them will have active recurring Crohn's within 5 years. For me, it was less than 5 weeks. The risks of it coming back can be reduced by taking medications. I was taken off all pharmaceuticals after my surgery, which I believe was a mistake.

About half of the patients who undergo surgery will need to have it again at some point.

I was surprised that the Crohn's and Colitis Foundation of America actually takes what I consider a balanced position regarding surgery and Crohn's disease on its website: "Many people suffer needlessly because they try to avoid surgery. But if medical therapy no longer keeps your disease under control, surgery should be seriously considered." And, "The combination of medical and surgical therapy can often give people with Crohn's disease the best possible quality of life."

A further, excellent recommendation is to optimize health via nutrition, exercise and meditation (being able to relax) prior to surgery. The healthier you are, the more likely that you will have a successful outcome along with a briefer recovery period.

Risks common to all surgeries include blood clots, heart attacks and infections, to name a few. That's why I believe each person with Crohn's must make the decision with his or her doctor. I would suggest researching which hospitals and surgeons have the best reputation. Your doctor is one possible source, but I have found that physicians were rather hesitant to recommend one surgeon over another. Nurses were a better source, as were non-medical members of the general population who were willing to share honest opinions. The Internet is another valuable tool for such information.

One of the decisions when having an operation is whether to undergo conventional or laparoscopic surgery. The former requires a 5- or 6-inch incision in the mid belly. The latter, which is done with a robotic device, is performed with four or five small incisions and possibly a 2- or 3-inch cut if the surgeon needs to get his or her hand inside your gut. Because it is not as invasive, patients spend less time in the hospital and recover more quickly. Laparoscopic surgery was not available to me when I had my ileum removed, but if I ever have need of more intestinal work, I will do everything possible to go that route.

Non-conventional Treatments

Commonly used alternative treatments for Crohn's are vitamin and mineral supplements, probiotics, fish oil and acupuncture. Medical websites and physicians will caution that these therapies have not been proven. Natural herbs and supplements may interact with medications or each other causing potentially serious problems. Even when taken alone, they may have side effects, and it is a good idea to inform your doctor that you are using them. Acupuncture or hypnosis have helped some Crohn's patients, but neither has been well enough studied regarding Crohn's disease to be conclusive and accepted by the medical profession.

Personally, I am convinced that alternative therapies have played a significant role in my ability to have a great life with Crohn's disease. I also believe that the reason they are not more widely accepted has to do with the way medicine currently works in the United States.

Since physicians are trained according to the scientific method, they generally don't accept anything but study-based evidence. I understand the importance of testing regarding medical therapies. However, most of them are conducted by the large pharmaceutical companies, that have a big incentive to do expensive scientific tests. When they can prove that a drug they have developed works, they will have a 20-year patent on the product. That means they can sell it at a huge markup, unless a competitor gets another product approved that is better.

It is estimated that it costs anywhere from $55 million to $2 billion to bring a drug to market. The drug companies tend to estimate high, of course, to justify their prices. For example, I am taking Asacol. My insurance company pays about $500.00 each month for that prescription. Another prescription I take no longer has the protection of a patent, and it costs $10 for a 90-day supply.

Alternative therapies do not warrant patent protection. Without the promise of a big payoff at the end, there is little incentive for the large drug companies to test them. And who else is going to spend millions of dollars to prove that a supplement or therapy works? The answer, nobody.

What I have done is investigate the alternatives, see if my doctor has any objections, and then tread with care. Based on my own experience, I am a firm believer in using fish oils, probiotics, and acupuncture, as well as vitamin, protein, fiber and mineral supplements. However, if someone claims to have been "cured" of Crohn's, and is touting a "miracle" product, I am very skeptical.

Over the years, there have been some changes in attitudes. Fish oil and the omega-3 fatty acids it contains is more respected in the medical community now than it was 2 or 3 decades ago. Yet there may be risks involved. A recent study found a link between prostate cancer and higher levels of omega-3 fatty acids in the blood.

Probiotics, such as yogurt and buttermilk, have been used for centuries in both eastern and western cultures to promote good digestion or to help restore the beneficial bacteria in the digestive tract after surgery or antibiotic use. My own digestive system functions better when I have 1/4 to 1/2 cup of organic yogurt each day. I tried probiotic capsules but never found the right one for me.

Vitamin and mineral supplements are also more accepted by the medical community. It is important to do your research because some of them are not well absorbed by a healthy gut, even less so by someone with Crohn's. I take a liquid vitamin and mineral supplement. I also use organic psyllium husk as a fiber supplement. I started with much less than the recommended dosage and increased it slowly. I now adjust the amount depending on how my gut is doing that day.

As a vegetarian, I know how important it is to get adequate protein. Most protein products are meat and dairy based. I take an organic rice protein powder. Others I know swear by tofu and other soy protein products.

Acupuncture, I believe, is a great tool for managing Crohn's disease. During certain treatments, I could feel energy moving to the diseased part of my gut. That only happened a few times, but based on how I felt afterwards, I am certain I benefitted from all of my treatments.

There are a wide variety of training programs for becoming a licensed acupuncturist, and it is taught as a legitimate discipline in a number of medical schools in the United States. My first acupuncturist, in California, was a registered nurse, an American who had studied in China. After I moved back to Tennessee, I found an acupuncturist who had been a doctor in China before immigrating to the United States. Both were great. Unfortunately, acupuncture is fairly expensive and most insurance carriers don't cover it. However, if you can afford it and find a qualified practitioner, I highly recommend checking it out.

To live with Crohn's it is important to understand the what, when, where, who and why of it. Knowing about various treatments, medicines and supplements available is critical, just as it is important to establish a good working relationship with your doctor. However, if you want to live well with Crohn's, you need to do more than that, and that is what the following chapters are about.

Chapter 3
POSITIVE ATTITUDE

Some years ago, at my Dad's funeral, I ran into a first grade classmate of mine who, it turned out, also had developed Crohn's disease. Because of our common background and common illness, I took extra time to talk with her. Unfortunately, when I met her, she was in poor spirits. I remember her pensive mood, her dejected body language, her tentative tone of voice and her unhappy words. I can't help wonder how her negative attitude, in contrast to my optimistic approach to life, affected our separate journeys. Sadly, she died in her early 60's. Thankfully, I am still going strong at 68.

Of course, this example is anecdotal, but there are a number of studies now that suggest a positive attitude has considerable impact on our health and longevity.

In 1973, thousands of elderly in Germany participated in a test that measured their feelings of well-being and pleasure; in other words, it gauged their attitude. Twenty-one years later, in 1994, the 300 that scored highest on the test were 30 times more likely to be well and alive than the 200 that had scored the lowest!

According to www.mayoclinic.com, the general health benefits of positive thinking are a longer life, less unhappiness or depression, fewer colds, better mental and physical sense of well being, less heart and cardiovascular disease and a greater ability to handle troubles and stress.

Much time and print have been devoted to positive attitudes in seminars, books, and websites on success. Besides improved health, benefits include greater happiness, more energy, greater inner power and strength, and the ability to inspire and motivate yourself and others. Difficulties are fewer, and when they occur, you are better able to deal with them. I also believe that life smiles more at you and that people will respect you.

There seems to be a number of traits associated with having a positive attitude, notably affirmative, constructive and creative thinking. Positive thinkers want to accomplish their goals and they expect success—they believe in themselves and in their abilities. They can be inspired and are able to maintain that inspiration. They tend not to give up and treat problems as blessings in disguise, always on the lookout for solutions and opportunities. They actually choose happiness and exude self-esteem.

One definition of a positive attitude is an optimistic mental outlook with regard to a fact or state of being. This is not just a matter of seeing the world through rose-colored glasses. Being optimistic means putting the most favorable construction upon actions and events or to anticipate the best possible outcome. This is different from being Pollyannaish, which is characterized by having an unrealistic, unreasonable or illogically cheerful and confident mindset.

For example, if you react to your diagnosis of Crohn's disease with a big smile, imagining that you are going to live your life exactly the way you always have and wanted to, that is Pollyannaish thinking. In contrast, with a positive attitude you'll anticipate having to make some changes so that you can and will have the best life possible, maybe even better than it was before getting this disease. People with a negative attitude are more likely to respond to the diagnosis with defeat and a belief that life is always going to be terrible, so they might as well give up.

Most Crohn's patients experience all three from time to time. One day, they may have a positive outlook, working on discovering and eating the best diet possible. Another day, they'll succumb to a negative attitude and stuff themselves with food they love, knowing it will make them sick. Still another day, they may be Pollyannaish and sign up for an adventure vacation in a third world country with no notion of how the local climate, cuisine and lifestyle will impact their disease.

I am convinced that cultivating a positive attitude has made an enormous difference in how my Crohn's disease has affected me. Hopefully, this chapter will give you a greater understanding of the importance and benefits of this approach to life, as well as tools to develop and nourish it.

General Outlook

So how does having a positive attitude impact someone with Crohn's disease? For myself, I accept that I have Crohn's and cannot change that. However, I have decided that it will help force me to live a healthier life. I tell myself that if I can cope with this disease, I must be a strong person, which increases my esteem and self respect. On the other hand, my limitations encourage me to stay humble. Anybody can run a race, but if I run with a handicap that no one can see and do well or just finish, that requires someone with character, especially if I do it with a big smile.

In addition, my chronic health challenge forces me to become more creative in my thinking. For example, I am going to develop healthier eating habits and the food is going to be not just more nutritious, but also more delicious than that of my former diet. This requires some effort on my part. So I start to learn about cooking, presentation of meals, and how to have fun in the kitchen with my wife or with guests. I used to watch TV or sit at the kitchen counter making conversation, while Colette put together our meals. Now, I participate more, and with some music on and maybe a bit of wine on the weekends, we have a blast. Sometimes, I prepare the whole meal myself. She appreciates it, and it makes me feel great to give her a break.

Accomplishing Goals

Another important trait of a positive attitude is setting goals and looking forward to accomplishing them. I was over 60 years old when I decided to run a 5K (3.1 miles) race. True, I was slim and athletic, but

I didn't like running or even walking at a brisk pace, and I certainly had never attempted a distance race. I don't know why I decided to run in a Thanksgiving turkey trot 5K, granted, I had started to walk and run a bit because I had borderline high blood pressure. Yet, I set it as a goal and accomplished it. Much to my surprise, it was a great experience, and I have since participated in several runs. Doing it makes me feel more positive about myself, about having Crohn's, and about life in general.

It doesn't matter whether your goal involves a physical test, such as lifting a certain weight at the gym, a mental challenge like publishing an article or book, or whatever other challenge you may choose, the positive approach is quite similar in all cases. For the sake of illustration, I'll elaborate on the 5K. For me, that race was a snap compared to writing a book.

The first step is to have a look at what you're in for. Let's say you've made the decision to run, and you tell your spouse or parent or loved one that you want to go and see a turkey trot. If they laugh or don't support you, go by yourself or get someone else to go along. You'll see young and old participants, some in great, and some in not so great, shape. I guarantee, watching all those people run or walk will inspire you. Start training, even if it means just walking around the house once. Pretty soon you will be walking around the block and then a mile and then 3 miles. Depending on your level of condition when you start, you may only walk the turkey trot, but if you want to run it, you can work up to that, too, and eventually conquer that 3.1 miles. The key is to want to accomplish that goal.

Expectations and Inspiration

Expecting success is another positive attitude trait. The summer after I graduated high school, I sold books door to door. Had I known how hard it would be, I probably would have opted to work in the shoe store where I had been offered a job, but my naivety and an excellent one-week sales course gave me a mindset of expecting success. I ended up earning enough in 3 months to cover all of my living expenses and saved $2,000.

Great accomplishment for a 17 year old! I could never have done it if I hadn't believed I could.

Related to expecting success is having trust in inspiration and believing that you can maintain it over time. Once I decided that yoga was important to me, I sustained my initial excitement by attending workshops, reading books about it, watching DVDs and occasionally getting together with people who also enjoyed practicing it. In other words, I kept the fire fueled.

Persistence and Dealing with Problems

One way I have learned not to give up is to think about how others who have faced much greater obstacles than me, kept going.

In 1941, when England was faced with what many thought certain, defeat by Adolph Hitler's Nazi war machine, Winston Churchill as British Prime Minister, gave a stirring speech. He said, "Never give in. Never give in. Never, never, never—in nothing, great or small, large or petty—never give in except to convictions of honour and good sense. Never yield to force; never yield to the apparently overwhelming might of the enemy." His words roused the population and Britain held out against overwhelming odds until the United States entered World War II.

Another way to move forward is to look at problems as a blessing in disguise. That isn't always as easy as it sounds. When I was young, I decided I wanted to be a helicopter pilot. I passed the mental and the physical exams, but failed the eye test, even though I had 20/20 vision. Instead of wings, I eventually got a pair of glasses. I was devastated. To make matters worse, my college roommate at the time was accepted and became an army helicopter pilot. Tragically, his Vietnam tour ended in a helicopter crash. Mine ended with me, glasses and all, being promoted to Captain, an assignment to beautiful Colorado Springs, my first choice for my final year in the army.

Of course many helicopter pilots returned from Vietnam and some convoy commanders—my job for a year—did not. However, the survival odds were in my favor. In addition, had I not become interested in becoming an army officer, I would probably have been drafted and spent my year in Vietnam as a clerk or a grunt, rather than in an interesting and challenging job. Now, 45 years later, I occasionally still get a little twinge of regret when I think of how close I came to doing something I really wanted to do. I also know I have a choice and can look at the positive aspects and results of those events.

Choosing Happiness and Believing in Yourself

Most people don't think that happiness is a choice, but it is. You can look out the window, see a brick wall, and tell yourself that you may not have the best view in the world, but you are happy to have an apartment. Besides, you'll have privacy and won't have to worry about a neighbor across the air shaft looking into your bedroom! When you notice negativity creeping into your thoughts, force them out of your mind by replacing them with good, positive alternatives, even if you have to really focus to make that happen.

Believing in yourself and your abilities is another positive attitude trait. It is important to know yourself. My first job after the army was as a public health director for the American Cancer Society. At the suggestion of my boss, I delivered a canned speech with slide show at my first presentation to a group of educators, and it bombed. It was embarrassing! To make matters worse, I had to go back the following day to the same group. Fortunately, I believed I could do better. I prepared half the night. The teachers cringed when they saw me again, but by the end of the session, I had them eating out of the palm of my hand! It is just as important for me to believe when Crohn's flares up that I will be better, and that putting in the necessary homework will make it so.

A related trait is the ability to display self-confidence and self-esteem. The actual act of standing and sitting with good posture will communicate to yourself and others that you are a person that has worth. There is a saying, "Fake it till you make it," but I don't like it because it is fundamentally cynical. I prefer to think of it as practice. If you act like you are important, you will begin to believe it and so will others. Over time, your sense of personal value will come naturally.

Being Proactive

My final positive attitude trait is to continue to look for solutions and opportunities. The point is not to wait for a problem to come along so we can fix it, but to anticipate future difficulties to avoid or take care of. The idea is to look for opportunities to tackle because we see that the world is filled with more possibilities than problems.

Steps to Developing a Positive Attitude

Even when we practice these traits, there is always room for improvement. The website www.successconsciousness.com recommends doing the following:

- choose to be happy and optimistic
- find reasons to smile more
- have faith in yourself and the power of the universe
- understand that negative thinking and worrying have negative results
- surround yourself with happy people
- read positive things
- memorize sayings that inspire and motivate you
- visualize only those things that you want to get
- learn to control your thoughts
- study concentration and meditation

In an article on the www.cbsnews.com website titled "Achieve a Winning Attitude in 6 Easy Steps," Geoffrey James suggests:
- understand you have the power to view anything and everything either positively, negatively or neutrally

- look at failures and setbacks in a constructive way
- feed yourself with positive thoughts and emotions through reading, movies, music, etc.
- avoid the news
- stay away from negative people
- use a positive vocabulary

I call them foundation blocks rather than steps because they don't have to be done in order. One or several can be used, but the more blocks you utilize, the stronger the foundation for a positive attitude.

Let's make our own list for developing a positive attitude, using the above and anything else that works. Remember, we have the power to see the world in the way we choose.

Choose to see life and the world as a wonderful and amazing gift

When it is cloudy, I appreciate how that puts a different tone on my environment. The cooler weather in the warm Florida climate is invigorating. I get to wear clothes that are a little different from the usual shorts and T-shirts. I know I am going to appreciate the sun even more when it pops out. I think about how dull it would be if our weather were always the same.

I realize that my Crohn's disease has shaped my life and made it more interesting. I have received many gifts along with its challenges. I often think about how the challenges of Crohn's have encouraged me to learn many new and wonderful skills.

Decide to be happy and optimistic

When I notice that I've let unhappiness or negativity creep in, I simply tell myself that I will be happy even if the situation is very challenging. I put a smile on my face, just to nudge my nervous system. Studies have shown that smiling changes one's mood. It's impossible to feel depressed when the corners of your mouth are turned upward.

Give yourself permission to have a bad day

Okay, I admit it. I'm not perfect. If I am having a negative day and I can't turn it around, I can surrender to it. The next day, I will redouble my efforts to be happy and optimistic. I try to figure out why I was in a funk and work to not let it happen again

Examine setbacks and failures to understand how to use them to your benefit

Let's say I am in a funk all day. I get up the next day. I don't feel great physically. Mentally I am down. I determine I don't need to see the doctor, but I decide to take a sick day and just work on myself. Aerobic training is out of the question. I do my meditation lying down instead of my usual sitting position. For breakfast, I take the time to fix the meal that I believe would be best for me. I take a short and slow walk. I listen to soothing and uplifting music. I read some positive quotes. Maybe I watch a positive movie or read an inspiring book. The idea is to do everything I possibly can to make myself feel better.

Watch and listen to more good stuff than bad stuff

I don't agree with never listening to the news. I believe awareness of our surroundings is important, even if it is not always pleasant. But I strive to live by the 3 to 1 rule, if I watch 30 minutes of news—most of which is negative—I need to counter it with at least 90 minutes of watching something uplifting.

If I read a book about factory farms for livestock (depressing), then my next book can be about growing an organic garden in the suburbs (uplifting). My next may be a historical novel, both educational and entertaining, my third any book that is a fun read for me. They are not always going to be in that sequence but over time I do try to keep a balance. To be realistic, if I watch 30 minutes of news, I probably won't watch 90 minutes of uplifting TV. So I have to come up with a plan to feed in at least 3 times more positive data to my brain and nervous system than negative data. If you watch or read something that is just fun and entertaining, that is great. But, if the entertainment has a negative flavor, such as sarcasm, then you have to counter it, just like with the news. Listening to music, watching an inspirational biography, reading a good self-help book all fit the bill. Sometimes, the news isn't negative, just trivial or silly. If I can laugh at it out loud, it makes a world of difference.

Speak and think in positive terms

I think of Crohn's disease as a challenge, not a problem. I don't "avoid junk food," I "strive to eat healthy food." Instead of thinking it is too hot to walk today, think I will exercise in the house today where it is nice and cool.

Exercise

I do yoga, walk, bicycle, kayak, paddleboard and more, but I recommend starting out with 10 or 15 minutes a day and working up to 30 to 90 minutes at least 5 days a week.

Spend time out of doors in nature and in the presence of physical beauty

I prefer to do my walking or running outside. Colette and I go sailing whenever we can, visit local parks regularly and go to state and national parks on our vacations.

If you live in a big city, parks and museums are great sources. If you live in the suburbs, find the closest good park. Travel a little farther for nicer ones on the weekends. Not many live in rural areas today, but if you do, find that special place or places to be with nature. The national parks are a great resource. Use them when you can. There are also some great county and state parks.

Meditate

For me, meditation is the best way I know to promote concentration, calmness and serenity. I know that there are some people who think it runs counter to their religion. Frankly, I think they are misinformed. I believe it enhances religious practice. I also believe some types of prayer can be a form of meditation.

Nourish your spiritual being

Like anything personal, this is an individual matter. For some, it may involve prayer or worship in a church, synagogue or mosque. For others, it may be exploring a set of beliefs unrelated to organized religion. Still others may find it uplifting to engage in activities that give their life a special meaning. So long as the spiritual practices are positive, embrace life, celebrate human kindness and inspire confidence, I believe that they are all spiritual practices well worth pursuing.

Accept that you will backslide from time to time

I have made a compact with myself that when it happens, I will forgive myself and find a way to recharge my optimism batteries with seminars, books, or anything that inspires.

Believe in yourself

For me, that is the most powerful tool of all. I keep telling myself that I can do whatever I want to do. I try to be realistic, but always strive for being the best I can be.

This may feel like an overwhelming project if you're trying to turn your life around, but if you start with one of these suggestions and see where it takes you, the process is manageable. Keep going by adding others and before you know, it will snowball and you'll never look back.

❧ *Chapter 4*
DIET

A friend's 25-year-old daughter was recently diagnosed with Crohn's and had to have surgery. After surgery, her doctor told her that diet did not affect Crohn's and to eat what she wanted. I heard the same from my doctors whenever one of my serious flare-ups was under control.

I mention this story because what I thought was old-fashioned, outmoded thinking, dismissing the importance of diet, still has a powerful hold on many physicians. As I have indicated earlier, my personal experience with the food I eat strongly suggests otherwise, and I believe more and more health providers, including medical doctors, understand that diet plays a significant role in coping with Crohn's. If your doctor believes otherwise, you may want to consider looking for another or simply use the information in this book and other sources to create the diet that is right for you.

If the purpose of our food culture were to promote the spread of Crohn's and other diseases, it would be considered very successful.

There are two reasons for that. One is that so much of our food is now processed. The other has to do with the way we raise the meat and vegetables we eat. Both have undergone dramatic changes in my lifetime.

I grew up on a small 100-acre farm in Tennessee, about 40 miles southeast of Nashville. When I was 4 years old, my dad received the "Farmer of the Year" award in Rutherford County. He was honored primarily because he had been the first in our county to have a state-of-the-art, grade "A" dairy farm. The "huge" herd of 35 cows was called, or driven, from the pasture into an old barn. Then a few of the animals were coaxed into a holding pen. From there, they were taken two at a time into a room with a concrete floor and feed troughs on each side of a pit. My dad would stand in the recessed pit, wash the cows' udders and apply automatic milkers to them. When they were finished being milked, he would open the doors and with a pat on the rump send the cows out into an open field.

If you're at all familiar with the history of farming in the United States, you know that this award-winning, state-of-the-art, 1950 dairy farm was obsolete within a decade. In the updated farms, 10 or more cows were being milked at a time. At that point, they still grazed on open pasture, but herds were growing larger. Because of the larger capital outlay for more advanced equipment, the herds grew larger and larger.

The story of what happened since then has been told in detail in other books. Two excellent reads are *Animal Factory* by David Kirby and *Fast Food Nation* by Eric Schlosser.

Suffice it to say, today there are factory farms in which the animals are kept in narrow pens and never see the light of day, instead of grazing on a grassy meadow, and some are even force fed. Almost all are fed grains and other food products, laced with growth hormones to "bulk" them up and make them grow faster. I don't know if that is why seven-year old girls are developing breasts before reaching puberty, but I know hormones can be powerful and dangerous.

The concentration of livestock, including cattle, chickens, pigs, etc., breeds disease, requiring them to have antibiotics administered. The process has become so repulsive that laws have been passed protecting our feed factories from having pictures taken of them.

Ignoring for a moment the damage these factory farms do to the environment and the inhumane way they treat the animals, why does this matter? The bottom line is that the change in the way our livestock is raised means that our food has changed, too. Some individuals and their intestinal tracts can cope with these changes just fine. Others, however, experience difficulties. Their bodies treat this food as substances from which they need to protect themselves. Their overreactions to the perceived danger set up an inflammatory, immune response, which in turn causes big health problems and, I am convinced, leads to many autoimmune diseases.

It is no accident that Crohn's and many other autoimmune disorders are almost non-existent in certain cultures while flourishing in others. In general, the less developed nations have significantly lower incidences of this disease, as well as rheumatoid arthritis, multiple sclerosis, asthma and psoriasis, than Western Europe and the United States. According to *Eating Right for a Bad Gut* by James Scala, Ph.D., there are certain countries and/or geographic areas that have almost no inflammatory bowel disease.

A case in point is the difference between Denmark and Greenland. Based on population studies done by epidemiologists and published in a 1980 Scandinavian medical report, the occurrence of Crohn's and other diseases was quite low, or almost non-existent in Greenland, but was quite high in Denmark. Besides Crohn's, the disorders included heart disease, diabetes, asthma, multiple sclerosis, rheumatoid arthritis, ulcers, breast cancer and other inflammatory bowel diseases.

I was surprised to learn that both populations ate a lot of fat, which Americans currently consider a dietary no-no. The Greenlanders got 39% of their calories from fat, the Danes 42%. The main difference was that the Greenlanders ate more food containing omega-3 fatty acids, which inhibit inflammation, while the Danes consumed more omega-6 fatty acids, which promote inflammation. In practice, the Danish diet consisted of more pork, red meat and saturated fats, while the Greenlanders' diet contained more fish and polyunsaturated fats.

The details are provided in Dr. Scala's book, and I would highly recommend that anyone with any inflammatory bowel disease, including Crohn's disease, take a look. I had to read it twice before it really sunk in.

The Omega-3 and Omega-6 Story

So, omega-6s are the culprits, right? No! Actually, they are just as important to our diet as omega-3s. Neither fatty acids can be manufactured by the body. They must be obtained from the food we eat, and both are essential to our well being.

As precursors to pro-inflammatory compounds, omega-6s are cellular components which produce inflammation. At one level, inflammation is good because it fights infection. The problem is, too much inflammation is not good. All the illnesses that end with "itis" such as arthritis, bursitis and ileitis are caused, in part, by too much inflammation. Also, cardiovascular disease, certain cancers, diabetes and even some mental health problems thrive in a pro-inflammatory setting.

Omega-3s, on the other hand, are the cellular component from which anti-inflammatory compounds are developed, and they encourage a healthy body environment.

Both fatty acids compete for the enzymes that convert them into biologically active compounds. If they are consumed in the right balance, they work "hand in hand" and do their job well. If there are too many omega-6s for every one omega-3, however, things tilt heavily toward excessive inflammation, which creates an unhealthy environment for the human body.

This problem occurs when we eat them in the wrong proportion. According to an October 2002 article "The Importance of the Ratio of Omega-6/Omega-3 Essential Fatty Acids" by A. P. Simopoulos, our earliest human ancestors probably had a diet with a 1 to 1 ratio of omega-6 to omega-3. However, the problem is that western diets today are about 16 to 1. The recommended ratio for healthy individuals is up to 5 to 1, and for individuals with disease, as low as 2 to 1. The bottom line is that no one benefits from eating at a 16 to 1 or greater ratio, especially if you have a disease exacerbated by inflammation such as Crohn's. Most of us will be better off increasing omega-3s in our diet and decreasing omega-6s.

Although beef or red meat is considered one of the bad omega-6 offenders, the problem is not beef per se, but the way most of it is raised. In the United States, almost all of the beef produced and consumed nowadays is grain fed, and has the unhealthy 20 to 1 ratio. Grass-fed or "free range" beef, on the other hand, has the more beneficial 4 to 1 ratio.

There is disagreement on the exact numbers of this ratio. However, every source I found confirmed that grain fed beef has a higher omega-6 to omega-3 ratio than grass-fed. While there is a "grass roots" movement to produce more traditional beef, it can't compete in price or quantity with the farm factories. Just go to your local supermarket and tally all the red meat in the cooler that is grass-fed or free range and compare it to the rest and you'll get the picture.

The same is true for eggs. Free range eggs have the more favorable 4 to 1 ratio, while regular supermarket eggs are about 20 to 1.

To get more omega-3 in your diet, eat wild, not farm raised fish, such as salmon and shrimp. Kale, broccoli, romaine lettuce, spinach and flaxseed oil are all good sources, as are kidney beans, although they may be hard to digest. I also use supplements—fish oil and chia seeds. Check with your doctor before taking either. With chia seeds, I started with a serving of one third of the recommended amount and worked my way up to one half. They tend to firm up my stool—a good thing for me—but sometimes, too much, which causes constipation—not so good.

To lower omega-6 in your diet, avoid most fast foods, corn oil, peanut butter, and foods with a high shelf life such as crackers and chips. Also avoid factory food. That includes processed foods—anything that comes in a box, can, or package and the contents look nothing like the original food. Factory food, also, is anything raised on a factory food farm. That means most eggs, milk, meat, poultry, and farm raised fish.

What to Do?

What does this mean as far as managing Crohn's disease? It means minimizing your factory food intake. The alternative is eating organic.

I always recommend doing so when it fits in the budget. Since reading *Tomatoland: How Modern Industrial Agriculture Destroyed Our Most Alluring Fruit* by Barry Estabrook, I almost never eat a tomato unless it is organic. For me, it has nothing to do with politics and is all about health. I believe buying organic is worth it, even if it costs more.

About 20 percent of people with Crohn's have a problem with bread and should strive to eat a gluten-free diet. For those suffering from Celiac disease, in which gluten leads to the destruction of their digestive system, it is literally a matter of life and death. If you are one of them, there are gluten-free breads, other baked goods, and flours available.

I love cheese but hardly ever eat it because it doesn't agree with me. The vegan substitutes I've tried, unfortunately, are not that great, in my opinion. I have settled on eating goat cheese. It is not available in all the varieties that cow cheese is, however, it is the real thing, can taste great, and doesn't bother my gut. I eat it in moderation.

If through trial and error you find that you have a problem with a particular food, eliminate it and look for a substitute.

Some readers of this book may consider starting an organic garden. They may also consider urban or suburban chicken and egg farming. If you do go this route, just remember that start up costs will be greater than you think, and it will require more work and commitment than you ever imagined. The best advice I can give is: start small. Not only is there work to raising and taking care of the garden or chickens, you have to either freeze or can or dehydrate your harvest. That takes work and planning. I would recommend staying away from it unless you have a passion for it.

Getting the Right Information

When gathering data about food, who can you trust? In my opinion, hardly anyone. That includes the government, the sellers and producers, and doctors or nutritionists. It's not that they deliberately peddle falsehoods. Many are well-intentioned folks who think they are telling the truth, but they've been sold a bill of goods and never checked their sources. There are some, unfortunately, who lie deliberately, just the way the tobacco companies used to about the dangers of cigarettes.

Take the U.S. Department of Agriculture's (USDA) food pyramid, recently turned into a "plate" with five different food groups—fruits, grains, vegetables and protein, and a small bowl of dairy on the side. I used to look at it as a good guide, but what I learned was that it changes with evolving beliefs about food and reflects the interests of certain powerful groups.

In November of 2011, for example, the U.S. Congress passed a bill declaring pizza a vegetable for what goes into school lunches because it contains a smear of tomato sauce. Food companies that produce frozen pizza for schools requested the change through their lobbyists. Does anyone think they really had the best interests of children in mind?

Food labels don't tell the whole story either. When looking at the "Nutrition Facts" on a store-bought product, 0% trans fats does not mean it has no trans fats, just less than 1% per serving. Once again, federal law permits labeling it so, even though it's like saying that a little sex never leads to pregnancy.

So what can you do to navigate the treacherous waters of our modern world of bad food and half truths if you have Crohn's disease? First, you have to believe good food is essential to your health. We are what we eat. Then, you have to do research by checking out books, websites and credible health providers—in general, any source not trying to sell you something. Fortunately, there are now a good number of them. My favorite is Scala's *Eating Right for a Bad Gut*. There is disagreement about some of his findings and recommendations, but I wouldn't let that stand in the way of benefitting from his expertise. My feeling about that is: Each "bad gut" is different and what is right for mine may not be right for yours.

Notice, I left off television. Some of what's on TV about food is accurate and truthful, but much of it is controlled by advertisers that have to sell you something to make a profit. In the process, they may do very well, but at your cost.

My Solutions

I am, primarily, a pescatarian, meaning I eat mostly grains and vegetables, fish, eggs and dairy, but no red meat, pork and fowl. I am not a zealot—I eat a little turkey occasionally, if it comes from a clean source. Turkey breast has a very high protein to fat ratio.

Water is my usual beverage of choice, but sometimes I will have a glass or two or three of wine, especially on weekends.

Typically, I eat three meals a day. Sometimes, I eat a mid-morning and a mid-afternoon snack. The key, I believe, is to eat less and to feel a little hungry, but not too hungry before eating again. To maintain a healthy gut, eating 2 to 3 hours before going to bed is fine. For me and others who digest slowly, 4 to 5 hours is much better. Don't eat breakfast until 12 hours have passed since your last food intake the night before. Finally, I have found that keeping to a consistent pattern works best. (More on specific menus and food items in the next chapter.)

One day on the weekend, my wife and I will eat out. We search for restaurants with the healthiest menus. Be aware that most restaurants cook with corn, cottonseed or soybean oil, all high in omega-6. If you get a greasy aftertaste from your pancakes, keep looking for a better place.

Shopping for Food

My philosophy about buying food is simple: Stay away from processed foods as much as possible. When purchasing processed foods, read the labels and choose the one with the shortest list of ingredients. Stay away from anything that has hydrogenated ingredients. Choose organic products as available and as your budget allows.

When it comes to vegetables in regular grocery stores, they are generally the tastiest and of the best quality when they are most plentiful and inexpensive because they are in season. It's the law of supply and demand.

I get as much food from farmer's markets as possible, being careful to buy from the local producers, not the vendors that buy from wholesalers. Often, the latter get their products from far away, including other countries. I like to get to know the local farmers and find out about their growing techniques. If they are not certified organic, do they at least limit their pesticides and what are they? Another important question is about surrounding farms that use pesticides. Sometimes a small grower grows organic but is not certified.

In many cases, frozen food may be healthier than fresh. It takes time to transport the food to market. If it is flash frozen, it may have more nutrients than the fresh version that has been deteriorating since it was picked or killed. Covering all bases, I eat some of both.

I eat wild caught salmon, and go for fish from more northern, less polluted seas. Two of my favorites are salmon and shrimp, both high in omega-3s.

Preparing Food

When I grew up, we ate most meals cooked at home. Since then, our culture has gone 180 degrees in the opposite direction. As a nation, we consume most of our food in restaurants and fast food places, convinced that preparing food is not a good use of our time and that we should pursue our careers instead, networking, socializing, facebooking, whatever. It's really just a choice to eat food prepared by others or by ourselves.

When I eat at a restaurant, I have no idea what I am eating. The wait staff has no idea what they are serving. Often, they think margarine and butter are the same. When I ask if the dessert whipped cream is real whipped cream, the server usually looks at me like I'm from another planet. I have learned to ask if the whipped cream comes from a can. If the answer is yes, I skip dessert.

What about prepared food from grocery stores that just needs to be heated or microwaved? The good news is that you can at least read the ingredients label, but do I really want to eat all that stuff that's listed—

often a lengthy paragraph of additives, coloring agents and preservatives? Very seldom. The bottom line for me is, I have decided it is worth my time (and health) to prepare my own food most of the time.

Luckily, I have a wife who likes to cook healthy, tasty meals. She has been cooking most of her life, but she also does a lot of research via cookbooks, the Internet and other sources.

Taking Colette out of the equation, how would I fare on my own? First, I'd buy two aprons, both looking manly, of course! (Joke!) One of the beauties of an apron is that you can wipe your hands on it when needed. It also helps put me in the mood to cook. After that, it's about starting small and getting some help from books or advice from a pro. If you mess up, keep trying. Watch how the cook on the brunch line prepares your omelet. It won't take long until you get all the steps right. So, dress for the job, focus on the job, start small, research as needed, and don't be afraid to make mistakes.

Trial and Error

I recommend a certain amount of adventurousness. Having to change your approach to food encourages you to explore things you may have never considered before. Try them and see if they work for you. If not, it's easy to eliminate them from your diet.

On Friday nights, Colette and I used to make homemade pizza. She'd prepare the dough and freeze it in individual balls earlier in the week. We'd thaw one for each of us and let them rise during the day. That evening, we made the pizzas together. We put on some music, shared a beer and talked about the day. Colette prepared the veggies and got the cheese out. My first job was to spread the dough and put it on the pan. I even learned to toss the dough but most of my spreading was on the cookie sheet—we liked our pizzas very thin. I put on the veggies and cheese and we popped our pies in the oven.

The problem was the cheese was a catalyst for my body to create mucous. After several challenging, sleepless nights, I decided to do without pizzas. The cheese was just too much for me. I listened to my body and made adjustments. After some trial and error, we found another meal we loved just as much. Since we like Indian food, we bought Indian food packets, naan bread, prepared basmati rice and some fresh vegetables to mix in with the Indian dish. Colette, always exploring healthy tasty meals, has learned how to make some excellent spinach paneer. I am a lucky guy.

Often on the weekends, we will have a dessert. Usually, it is homemade. If I eat ice cream, which is not good for me, I try to eat it early in the day so the mucous subsides by bedtime.

I have also discovered an ice cream substitute, which I think is great—coconut milk ice cream. A pint costs more than a half gallon of regular ice cream. I tell myself that eating less is good for the waistline. By the way, studies show brains shrink as waistlines expand.

Special Events and Holidays

Food rituals around all-American events and holidays are almost like sacred cows in India—don't touch them! Woe to those who disregard tradition. In some families and social groups, they are treated like lepers. For someone with Crohn's, that presents a special challenge.

One year, we were invited to a neighborhood Super Bowl party. The game started about 6:30 p.m., and the party, two hours earlier. Because it was Monday and we were working, we arrived at 5:45. We said our hellos and were guided to the food table. The spread included chicken wings, meatballs, chips, shrimp with cocktail sauce on the side, artichoke dip, and a taco-flavored cream cheese dish, among others. We had already reminded the hostess we were vegetarian plus fish eaters. I have always done fine with shrimp and cocktail sauce, so I had a few chips with artichoke dip; but the item that caught my attention was the cream cheese, sour cream, mango, black beans, red pepper, cilantro dish and taco mix seasoning that was to be eaten with corn chips. "Lucky" for me, there was more than enough of it to go around, and I indulged.

When halftime came around, we said our goodbyes as the others were finishing up their cowboy stew. Nobody seemed to care much that we were not meat eaters.

I find it has become easier over the years to fit in at parties with a Crohn's disease diet. I think this is due in part to a changing culture, but mostly because of my own strategies and my acceptance that I am going to have to be a little different. Some people never get it and think my diet is some sort of political statement, while others respect that I have the strength to eat as I need to. Some seem flustered by it and make awkward jokes or statements, while others ask intelligent questions about why I eat the way I do and about the food culture as a whole. Most just want to enjoy what they are eating.

My favorite strategy for dealing with party food is to eat before I go and just politely nibble on the few things I've put on my plate before tossing them in the garbage. If I find something that fits my diet and I really like it, I have saved a little stomach room and enjoy it. But most of the time, I just make the event or the people my focus rather than the food.

Sit-down dinners with friends or relatives are tricky. I find it easier to be a vegetarian who eats fish. However, this is not a sure bet. On one occasion, we were served tuna, raw vegetables, a salad and chocolate dessert. The hostess was already flustered, hers being a meat and potato family. Imagine her look when I sheepishly informed her that I was allergic to tuna and chocolate, and that raw vegetables did not work for me. Luckily, there was some bread and butter in the house, and we all survived the evening. Since then, Colette and I are more specific ahead of time about what we can and can't eat, and maybe as a result, we are seldom invited to a sit-down dinner.

Surprisingly, I usually do quite well at potluck meals. There is enough variety that I often find several dishes to my liking, which also like me. Usually, what I eat is not the most popular food on the table, so there is almost always enough for seconds if I want more.

Cookouts are another thing, however. They usually consist of hamburgers, hotdogs, potato chips, and gloppy coleslaw. Colette and I usually bring a fillet of salmon and do fine. If you are a vegetarian, learn how to grill tofu. It can be quite tasty with a good sauce.

When it comes to holidays and anniversaries, things can go either way. We often indulge, but try to keep the bad stuff to a minimum. For example, on my last birthday, we went to a Greek restaurant at the beach and except for an extra glass of wine, ate a very healthy meal. However, on Colette's birthday we went to a different restaurant that serves heavenly fried oysters. I ordered a plate of them, as well as hushpuppies and coleslaw. At least I passed up the French fries. I felt it afterward, but by having lunch instead of dinner and following up our overindulging with a bike ride, I did okay.

As for holidays, I almost wrote a chapter on Thanksgiving because it symbolizes the good, the bad and the ugly of our relationship with food, but I will keep things brief. Personally, I love the two big holidays, Christmas and Thanksgiving, best of all. In many ways, my favorite is Thanksgiving because it is the less demanding of the two. But let's admit it, the focus for most of us is not about being thankful for what we have, but on the meal, which presents us with difficulties.

I will eat turkey on Thanksgiving, but that is not the major problem for me. It is overeating. I admit that there have been times when I have thrown caution to the wind, binged on the delicious spread of some of my favorite foods, and suffered the consequences that night and the next day.

However, rather than beat myself up, I remember that there will always be times like this. When I overeat, I try to keep moving. If that is too challenging, I sit up. If sitting up is too challenging, I sit in a reclined position of about 60 degrees (absolutely not less than 45 degrees). Remembering my motto, "All things in moderation, even moderation," I accept that I have splurged on the "even moderation" portion for a day. To get back on track, I pull out my recipes and meal plans, and that brings us to the next chapter.

Chapter 5
MEAL PLANS AND RECIPES

Since discovering that the primary key to managing my Crohn's disease is to control my diet, my wife or I cook most of my meals. In that regard, I have been on the outside of normal, current eating habits. Some may describe me as a retronaut—who likes to rummage around in the past—others may call me a visionary. I think of myself as a pragmatist, although I like to think that I have been anticipating ideas, practices and attitudes that are finally beginning to make their way into mainstream American consciousness.

For example, best selling food author, Michael Pollan, argues in his 2013 book, *Cooked*, that we should get back to preparing nourishing foods ourselves, rather than leaving it up to corporations to supply us with processed foods or restaurants to give us meals laden with noxious oils and salt. It is perhaps the most significant step we can take to improve our health, our family relationships, and even our link to the natural world. I couldn't agree more.

The key is to make the experience of reclaiming our kitchens enjoyable. With that in mind, here are some of my favorite recipes.

Breakfast Ideas

Vegan milk

I prefer the nondairy milk found in the refrigerated section of the supermarket. Low fat soy (more protein) is my favorite, but almond or coconut milk also work. The non-sweetened versions are great and contain less sugar. If I am going camping or want a backup at home, I get the kind that does not need refrigeration until it is opened, although it is more expensive, not as tasty, and has more preservatives in it than I prefer. The low fat variety is my choice because soy products have a high omega-6 to omega-3 fatty acid ratio.

Coffee

I buy organic French roast beans that I get at the grocery store. I grind them myself in an inexpensive little grinder and then put through a drip coffee maker with a natural paper filter. The drip filter system, according to an article I read in The New York Times, removes the part of the coffee bean that raises cholesterol. I like my Joe strong with a third to half cup of soy milk, heated in the microwave.

Oatmeal

I eat mine with butter or vegan substitute, banana, soy milk and sweeteners like agave nectar or honey. Take

> 1/3 cup oatmeal
> 2/3 to 1 cup of water

and boil them together on the stove until ready—about 5 minutes—stirring as often as needed so it does not stick. I like my oatmeal well done.

Cheerios®

Okay, they are a processed food and not ideal, but if I am in a hurry or lazy, they are a good option and they don't leave me with any ill effects. I eat them with soy milk, sometimes with bananas or frozen peaches. They are one of my "comfort foods."

Health drink

Take

- 8 ounces of orange juice (for a smoothie-like consistency) or 8 ounces of low fat soy milk (for milk shake-like consistency)
- 8 ounces of water
- 1/2 to 1 whole banana
- 1/3 to 1/2 serving of fiber (whole husk organic psyllium)
- 1 serving of brown rice or soy protein
- 1/4 to 1/2 cup French vanilla yogurt
- 1 serving of liquid multi-vitamin and mineral supplement

Mix in a blender, pour into a glass, and drink. I often use this after a good run or workout. To me, it tastes great and healthy. Recently I have been adding 1/2 serving of white chia seeds.

Eggs and faux sausage with biscuits, bagel or toast

Eggs can be poached, fried in canola oil, or scrambled. For the latter, I mix in a tablespoon or two of soy milk or water and often, chopped up cooked faux sausage. I use about 1/4 a serving of Gimme Lean® Sausage, a vegetarian, "meat" product.

Sometimes I have a peeled organic tomato slice or two on the side. I either peel the individual slice with a knife or to peel the whole tomato, drop in boiling water for 30 seconds, then dip into cold water from the tap. The peel comes off easily. If you want to remove the seeds, slice it into 1/4 or 1/8 sections lengthwise and with clean hands, take the seeds and excess water out of the tomato. Be sure to do this over the sink, or slice and remove peels on a cutting board.

Biscuits

Here is my biscuit recipe. If you are not from the South, you will probably want toast or a bagel, but here it is anyway. Try it, you just might love it.

I like to use white whole wheat flour because the results are more like traditional biscuits, but just as healthy as those made with less mild tasting whole wheat. The King Arthur non-organic brand is available at my grocery store. There is considerable variety among brands, so I recommend trying different ones until you find one you like. If I want lighter biscuits, usually for company, I mix one cup of unbleached white with one cup of white whole wheat.

Take

2 cups of flour

2 1/2 teaspoons of baking powder (I use low sodium, aluminum free)

1/2 teaspoon of salt (I use sea salt)

Mix these ingredients together with a fork and spread a couple of tablespoons of the flour mixture on the cutting board.

Then take

1 tablespoon of white vinegar

3/4 cup of soy milk

1/3 cup of extra virgin olive oil (You can use other oils such as canola, if you wish)

Stir the liquid ingredients together with a fork. Pour the result into the mixture of dry ingredients and blend. Add more soy milk if necessary. It is better to be a little too moist than a little too dry.

Place the resulting dough on a wooden cutting board that has been dusted with flour to keep it from sticking. Put more flour on top to prevent your hands from sticking to the dough and press down until flat and about 1/2 inch thick. Then fold over to get out the "wrinkles" Press down from two to five times until it is smooth. The fewer times, the better.

Cut out biscuits with biscuit cutter or small glass rim. Fold the leftover dough as before and repeat process. Remember, the biscuits do not have to look perfect to taste great.

Place the biscuits in one or two oiled cooking pans. I like Pyrex glass ones; they seem to cook more evenly than metal pans.

Cook in a preheated oven at 475 degrees for about 12 minutes.

Take out and put the ones you are going to eat in a covered dish, slightly cracked to keep them from getting soggy; or place them in a bowl in a tea towel. I put the others on a plate to cool. If you leave them in the hot pan, it may overcook the bottom.

Put the ones you did not eat in a freezer bag and freeze. We almost always freeze our leftovers. It works for 90% of the food we prepare. I usually eat two or three when fresh, but pull out only one from the freezer and microwave about 23 seconds for later meals.

Omelets

I am a great fan of omelets. Here are three of my favorite dishes.

Rice, faux sausage, and egg

Break "sausage" into small pieces while cooking in a skillet. Mix cooked rice and egg and browned "sausage" in a bowl. Salt and pepper or use a substitute seasoning to taste. In a frying pan, heat one tablespoon or so of canola or other oil. Pour mixed ingredients into pan and cook on medium high until brown on bottom. Flip over and cook till brown. A larger pan promotes faster, thorough cooking and a thinner omelet, which is my preference. Note: I usually use brown rice because it is more healthy, but I use white rice when my digestive system is a little off or I am in a hurry.

Grated potato, faux sausage and egg

This mixture takes more time to cook because the potato goes into the mixture raw. The rice, in the previous recipe, was already cooked. First peel, then grate one small to medium potato. This dish requires a large skillet. You don't have to cook the faux sausage as long, since it will get plenty of heat in the potato and egg mixture.

Chopped vegetables with or without cheese

In very light oil, sauté any combination of chopped vegetables. One of my many favorite combinations includes onions, red cabbage, and broccoli. It is important to pick vegetables that you digest well. Many have trouble with onions. I find as long as they are not greasy, and I eat a moderate amount, they go down very nicely.

Make sure the vegetables are chopped into small pieces, well cooked, and not too many. Combine egg, vegetables, and seasoning, mix with a fork, and pour into an oiled skillet. After flipping, put a little cheese or cheese substitute in the center. Fold in half and cook on both sides.

Counting the health drink as a meal, this provides seven or more ideas for breakfast.

Mid-morning or Mid-afternoon Snack

I only eat this when needed. If I have had a full breakfast or plan to have an early lunch, I will skip this snack and have it in the afternoon.

Health drink modified

Depending on what I have had for breakfast, I might drink 4 oz. of orange juice with rice or soy protein powder and fiber. I'll add everything except the banana and use less yogurt. Sometimes I substitute vegan milk for orange juice. You will just have to experiment with what works best for you. Bananas are my staple, but I also use peaches, blueberries or strawberries.

Peeled apples and soy "peanut" butter

Substitute almond butter if needed or desired. Because of my Crohn's, I have learned to always peel the apple. I already knew about peeling the bananas.

Yogurt with fruit and granola or crumbled graham cracker

I like organic French vanilla yogurt, which has a little sweetness. My wife prefers plain yogurt for most things.

Lunch

Tofu squares

Tofu is a white, solid but soft cheese-like product made from soybeans that comes in large cubes. Although it doesn't have much taste, it is a good source of protein, and okay when baked and doctored up with sauces and consumed with rice, or a baked potato and steamed vegetables.

For tofu squares, wrap one package extra firm tofu in cloth. Squeeze out water. Cut into eight slices. Drizzle, mix and coat bottom of a 9 x 13 Pyrex dish with one tablespoon of dark sesame oil, one tablespoon of Tamari (soy sauce) and one teaspoon of Mrs. Dash® Garlic & Herb seasoning. Place tofu slices in dish, coat one side and flip over. Bake at 350 degrees for 60 to 80 minutes or until golden brown. Cool completely to room temperature, place in zip lock bag and freeze.

TLT—Tofu, lettuce and tomato sandwich

Just like a BLT but with tofu instead of bacon. A thin slice of my favorite goat cheese makes it tastier. Consider using vegan mayonnaise, but carefully compare ingredients with your regular brand to make sure it is worth the extra cost.

Salmon sandwich

Mix a serving of wild canned salmon with sweet pickle relish and mayo (both are optional). For a healthier recipe, substitute a nourishing pesto sauce or salsa. Then add any or several of the following: lettuce, peeled tomato, spinach, peeled and de-seeded cucumber. Other greens or cabbage may be substituted for the spinach.

Chop or grate as desired. If my digestive system is acting a little sensitive, I steam or sauté the spinach in water and use it with the pickle relish and mayo or pesto or salsa with peeled and seeded tomato.

Place on whole wheat or multi grain bread and enjoy with or without a serving of baked chips. It is hard to eat one serving of chips, unless you count them out and close the bag and put the bag away. Okay, I usually count out two or three extra for good measure. Wean yourself off the chips for a healthier diet. Better yet, keep them out of the house.

Salmon salad

Same as above with or without brown rice mixed in. I eat it with or without crackers. If I don't include the rice, I may have a rice cake instead of the crackers. I put the extra servings of salmon in four or five individual baggies and put them inside another baggie for the freezer. One serving doesn't take long to thaw or prepare in the microwave if in a hurry.

Soup with brown rice and tofu chunks

I like to cut up tofu squares and add to my soup for protein and I enjoy crackers or cornbread on the side. If my digestive system is more sensitive on a particular day, I have tomato soup or any other soup that's not chunky, and I may use white instead of brown rice. If you are eating clam chowder or chicken noodle soup, the tofu pieces are not needed.

Hummus

Originally a Mediterranean dish, hummus is an excellent protein source made from chickpeas (also called garbanzo beans), tahini (sesame paste) and spices. It makes for a great lunch, spread on bread, crackers or vegetables, and I find it easy to digest. There are a number of ready-to-eat brands available in supermarkets. They come with different flavorings. My favorite is roasted red pepper. If you want to save money, make your own. It will be a lot less expensive and probably have better ingredients.

Dinner

Dinner is considered the principle meal of the day. When I grew up in Tennessee, the noon meal was referred to as dinner when it was the big meal of the day. If we had a light meal, it was lunch. The evening meal in my home was always supper, whether it was light or the main meal, but I will call it dinner for the purposes of this chapter.

Some research suggests the European way of consuming the main meal during the day, with a longer "lunch hour," is a healthier way of eating. For someone with Crohn's, I believe it is essential to eat the evening meal early and to keep it light. If I finish about 4 hours before I go to bed, I am more likely to sleep well and wake up with good energy and a healthy appetite in the morning. If I eat too much or too late, I pay the price the next day.

During the week, Colette and I keep our meals light. On the weekends, we eat a little more and a little later. However, we also stay up a little later on weekends. It works out pretty well.

Spinach and egg dinner

This one is really easy. Steam or water sauté fresh spinach. Medium-soft boil one or two eggs per person. Prepare some corn bread. The standard recipe is 1 cup flour to 1 cup corn meal. The flour can be unbleached white, white whole wheat (my favorite) or whole wheat. Use brown rice vinegar on spinach to taste. Serve with your favorite beverage. I like mine with a glass of wine.

Recently, I have learned to sauté with water instead of oil. I love it because it is healthier and the vegetables are easier for me to digest. This website explains how it is done: *http://healthygirl-skitchen.blogspot.com/2010/04/great-strategy-healthy-water-saute-ing.html*

Fish, fowl or other meat, potato and veggie

Another easy one. My choice is fish, caught wild from cold water such as the North Pacific or Atlantic Oceans. My favorite is salmon. If you want fowl, use free range and be careful of your source; if beef, use grass-fed, free range.

A serving the size of the palm of your hand is about right. Simply top with butter, oil and your favorite seasoning and place it in an oven-safe bowl and bake at 350 degrees until done. Check after 10 minutes, again after 5 minutes and then every 2 minutes, however long it takes to cook it. It takes a little practice. A fillet of salmon usually takes from 15 to 20 minutes. I like it well done, but if it is overcooked it will get tough.

To bake a potato, simply microwave for about 5 minutes or bake in oven at 350 degrees for about an hour. For your veggie, use fresh or frozen and cook until done to your liking. Serving with bread is optional.

Indian dinner

As I mentioned in the previous chapter, this is our Friday night dinner. It is fast, healthy and very tasty.

First, we cook 1/2 cup of white or brown basmati rice. Then we get a precooked, frozen or sealed package of an Indian dish and steam or sauté a fresh vegetable that complements it. We mix them together in a pot and cook them until the vegetable is no longer moist.

For bread, I take naan, an Indian bread that can be bought in most supermarkets, coat it with chopped or pressed garlic in melted butter, and heat it in the oven. Our only side dish is a mango or peach chutney. The dinner is served over the rice.

Beans

Beans are a great health food, but many with Crohn's have problems digesting them. I don't, however, and assume there are others who can eat them as well. If you are not sure, start with very small portions, say a teaspoon or so. If you take them from a can, drain and rinse them three or four times. Let them sit in the water for 10 or 15 seconds each time; then heat until they are a little mushy.

If you determine that you can eat beans, consider trying dry beans, soaked and cooked. Why not just buy canned beans? Because preparing your own dried beans is healthier and cheaper.

The easiest way is in a slow cooker. After soaking overnight, rinse several times, put the beans in a slow cooker, cover with water and cook on low for 5 to 8 hours. When you do this the first time, make sure you are at home to find out about how long it will take. They are done when they start to split and are easy to chew. Cooking them a little longer makes them easier to digest. Drain most of the water. Freeze what you don't eat in individual servings.

I usually cook two cups of dried beans at a time. Before you start, be sure to check the beans for little rocks. You don't want to bite down on one of them unsuspecting. Pour a few beans in a bowl and look for little pieces of gravel before putting them in the pot.

There are lots of different kinds of beans, including white, navy, black, lima or pinto beans, my favorite. Be careful of kidney or red beans; they are harder to digest. Lentils and other small beans take less time to cook. I am not wild about lentils, but my wife loves them. You may also.

Beans, rice, and greens

Steam the greens until they are well done. I like chard and beet greens and they do not take long to cook. Serve them with a little vinegar. Brown rice vinegar is less tart than balsamic or regular.

I like some chopped onions and sweet pickle relish in my beans. I mix them with brown rice and have the greens on the side. Organic peeled tomatoes go with this combination.

Dirty rice with beans

Cook faux sausage. Chop it up while cooking. Sauté some onions in canola oil. Put beans, the browned faux sausage and the onions in a pot. Heat and serve.

Drinks

My beverage for lunch is almost always water with a slice of lemon. In fact, I stick with water most of the time.

Sometimes, I will have a glass or two of wine, especially on weekends. I like dry wines and typically drink red, which is supposed to be good for the heart, but the jury is still out on that. I sleep a little better when I drink red wine. That may be because it typically has less sugar than the whites.

Summary

This is a week's worth of recipes—enough to get you started. Once you're on your own, don't worry. There are many great cookbooks out there, some specifically geared toward Crohn's disease. In addition, there are a bunch of TV cooking shows, and of course there is the Internet. I have found, as a result of having Crohn's, that I have expanded my range of foods and cuisines, which has been a lot of fun. If you approach cooking for yourself with joy, curiosity and imagination, you can't go wrong.

Chapter 6
EXERCISE

When I was 55, I attended a Crohn's seminar. As part of the activities, we had the opportunity to get screened for osteoporosis, loss of bone density being one of the many complications of the disease. I tested in the "good" range for a normal 27-year-old! The screener was amazed when I told her that I had been diagnosed with Crohn's 20 years earlier. I was pleased with the results and attributed them to my passion for exercise and sports.

Some years later at my dad's funeral, a woman approached me—we had gone to the same grade school together. She also had Crohn's disease. We talked briefly about our common challenges. She mentioned she had heard that I exercise a great deal. She didn't. I am sorry to say that she died 2 years later in her early sixties, about the same time I entered my first 10K run (6.2 miles). I didn't finish very high, but I was still "in the race."

I don't know the specific circumstance of her death, and can't say for certain that it came earlier because she didn't exercise, but given the way Crohn's affects the body, I believe staying physically active is essential, and I am convinced that it has helped me immensely and has been a major factor in improving the quality of my life.

I also believe that everybody can exercise. I will go as far as to say I believe everybody must exercise. Exercise is beneficial and necessary, not only to the bones and muscles, but to all the systems of the body including the brain and the digestive system. So whether you get winded walking to the mailbox or won the local turkey trot 5K, I would encourage you to develop and implement an exercise routine that will both challenge and nurture you.

Exercise and Crohn's Disease

Exercise can help mitigate many of the side effects of having Crohn's, including stress, funky moods and depression, fatigue and lower self-esteem. It turns out that working out regularly is an excellent antidote for all of them. Exercise also promotes a better body image, better memory and better cognitive function, and I'll bet it lowers the risk of Alzheimer's. Working out is a great way to strengthen bones. The benefits of exercise in combating osteoporosis, which affects everyone getting older, are especially more crucial for people with Crohn's.

Other advantages include improved skin, faster healing, tooth loss prevention, better balance, and optimum brain function. Above all, working out boosts weakened autoimmune systems, which is great news for people with Crohn's.

I must admit that I get somewhat frustrated when I read about specific studies and recommendations regarding Crohn's disease and exercise. They are too spotty and timid in their approach. Perhaps as someone with an athletic bent, my expectations were too high. Unlike other areas of medicine, there just hasn't been much research on the subject. Fortunately, the benefits of exercise for improved health and better lifestyle, in general, have been examined and verified. The bottom line is exercise may not make you live longer, but it will greatly improve the quality of the life you have.

Of course, it is important to consult your doctor before starting a new exercise program to find out what you can and can't do. But, in line with the meager research, it has been my experience that physicians don't always encourage those of us who are motivated to push ourselves as far as we can possibly reach. Part of the reason is that doctors are focused on medicine. They have spent years studying and practicing medicine and are used to prescribing pharmaceuticals to deal with their patients' ailments. Unless they are passionate about exercise themselves, they will not have the experience or wherewithal to make informed recommendations. So if your doctor seems too timid, you may want to consult another one or seek the advice of a professional trainer or physical therapist.

In Practice

Each of us has a different capacity for exercise, but everyone has the ability to exercise in some way. Some will need to have a modest routine, while others can, and will, pursue ambitious training. The challenge is to find a routine that is right for you and then figure out how to best weave it into the fabric of your daily life.

The beauty of exercise is that you can benefit from it very quickly. It doesn't matter if you are in bad shape. Unless you are suffering from a debilitating disorder or are physically incapacitated, you should be able to engage in some form of physical activity and reap its benefits.

After I had surgery to remove 3 ½ feet of my small intestine because my Crohn's disease had gotten so bad, I didn't want to do much more than lie in bed and watch TV. The nurses wouldn't have it. One of the first things I had to do was to sit up. Yes, sitting up in bed can be a challenging exercise. Soon after, they wanted me to walk to the bathroom, then down the hall. I tried to resist, but when they told me that if I didn't, I would get bed sores or pneumonia or worse, I grudgingly complied, and found I could do it with little difficulty. My point is that no matter how low we get in spirit, we can still exercise. We just have to find the type that is right for us at that moment.

For people with Crohn's, the most basic exercise program would consist of walking or riding a bike. However, if your disease is under control, you may be able to do much more. I have become a great fan of kayaking. I love being on the water, and I can go at a brisk or gentle pace, depending on what I feel like.

I am also a great advocate of running, but if you can't, or just don't want to do that, brisk walking or power walking is the best substitute. You can use a treadmill, but I prefer running or walking outside and believe that is more beneficial.

Good running gear is important. For over a year now, I have been using Vibram FiveFingers® footwear—the "shoes" are like gloves, providing separate places for each toe. As a result, I have had less knee pain and stiffness than in the past. I also really like the feeling—they are the closest thing to barefoot running and still having protection for the feet.

If you want to read up on the pros and cons of running footwear, as well as running in general, a good source, both entertaining and informative, is *Born to Run* by Christopher McDougall.

If in poor condition, here is a way to get started:

Week 1

Day 1: Walk around the outside of the house once.

Day 2: Walk around the house twice.

Day 3: Walk around the house three times.

Day 4: Walk one block and return or take a day off from exercise.

Days 5 and 6: Walk one block and return.

Day 7: Rest. You earned it. Pat yourself on the back.

Week 2

Days 1 to 6: Walk 2 blocks and return. That is almost 1/2 mile.

Day 7: Rest.

Week 3 and beyond

Walk about 10% further each week until you're walking up to 2 miles at a fairly brisk pace. That will take about 35 to 40 minutes.

Congratulations! You are now ready to go to the next level.

If you are severely overweight or have serious joint problems, this plan may not work for you. Participating in water exercise classes or using equipment like an elliptical machine at the gym, which does not stress the joints, may be the answer. But remember, osteoporosis is one of the complications of Crohn's disease and to counter it, requires stress on the bones. Consult your doctor and/or explore with a licensed physical therapist how to best deal with your joint or weight challenge to accomplish that. Wellness centers that partner with hospitals are usually a good place to get started. They are often expensive, however, so if you are on a budget, consider going for a few months, learning all you can, and then doing it on your own. If you are financially challenged, sometimes they will adjust the charges.

Different Types of Exercise

There are four basic types of exercise:

- Aerobic
- Core work
- Resistance training
- Stretching and flexibility training

We need all four.

Aerobic exercise

Any activity, which increases the body's demand for oxygen and in turn raises the respiration and heart rate, is considered aerobic. The best are running, swimming, brisk walking or biking, and aerobic classes. Sports such as singles tennis, soccer, racquetball and basketball are great, too, but they can be hard on the joints as we get older. To get aerobic benefit, you have to keep the heart and respiration rate up for 20 to 60 minutes no matter which activity you choose.

Aerobic exercise leads to the production of new capillaries in the muscles, the heart, and the brain, which increases the flow of nutrients and the removal of toxins. It also raises the number of circulating red blood cells, which improves the transport of oxygen, and causes blood vessels to produce nitric oxide, a relaxant that increases blood flow.

In addition to improving the efficiency of the body's cardiovascular system in absorbing and transporting oxygen, aerobic exercise also improves heart and brain function. Scientific studies have shown that it lowers the risk of heart attack and heart disease. It also lowers the risk of diabetes, stroke, obesity, osteoporosis, hypertension, gallstones, diverticulitis and many types of cancer. It relieves depression and actually reverses memory loss that happens as we age. Vigorous aerobic exercise may be the best "wonder drug" that exists.

For people with Crohn's, one of the special benefits is improved digestion. Aerobic exercise brings greater blood flow to the gastrointestinal tract which leads to an increase in intestinal contractions and digestive enzymes, mitigating constipation and other gut problems.

Core work

Referring to the center of the body—the stomach area front and back from the groin to below the shoulders—core exercises include sit-ups for the abdominals and "superman" exercise for the back. They improve balance, stability, and our overall ability to perform most physical activities with greater efficiency, whether it is reaching or bending. Stronger back and abdominal muscles make everything, from taking out the garbage, to picking up a child or grandchild, to swinging a golf club, both safer and more enjoyable. Core exercise is very important in preventing injury in our everyday lives.

There are several disciplines that deal specifically with core work, such as Pilates and The Feldenkrais Method®, as well as using an exercise ball, which can be done on an individual or group basis. There are

DVDs for those wishing to try them at home, but in my view, classes led by professional practitioners are best.

For the more adventuresome, try stand up paddle boarding. It improves balance as well as core muscles, and is a blast if you like water activities.

Resistance training

A type of exercise that uses weights or applied muscular pressure to one's own body to make muscles work or contract, resistance training builds strength, size and endurance of muscles. According to the Mayo Clinic, it will preserve and enhance muscle mass, develop strong bones, control weight, boost stamina, help manage chronic conditions, and even sharpen one's ability to focus.

Resistance training can be done on gym machines or with free weights. Most gym memberships come with a free session or two with a trainer who will explain and help you get to know the equipment.

It is now recommended by most health professionals that we do resistance training, such as weight lifting, as long as we live. Without it, the body becomes frail. Resistance training improves and maintains muscles and bones. It is particularly helpful in preventing osteoporosis. Running, walking, and biking all counteract the ensuing loss of bone density, but only weight training will do so for arms and spine.

If you run and don't do anything for the upper body, you are strong from the waist down and weak from the waist up. Does that make sense? Of course not. After age 50, we lose about half a pound of muscle per year. With weight training, we are able not only to stop that loss, but to increase the muscle mass in our body. Studies show that the earlier you start with weight training, the better, but no matter when you start, whether at age 16 or 86, you will reap benefits. Of course, remember to start with very light resistance and increase gradually.

Stretching and flexibility

These types of exercises lengthen a specific muscle or muscle group and improve elasticity, flexibility and circulation. Without flexibility exercises, we gradually lose our range of motion. Contracting muscles without taking time to lengthen or stretch them can strengthen them but does not allow them to function optimally. As everyone ages, due to many reasons, the connective tissue in the body binds together in an unhealthy way. Stretching prevents that and can correct it. Flexibility and optimum range of motion of our joints protects us from certain types of injury as well as allows us to do things we otherwise would not. More of this will be discussed in the next chapter on yoga.

Specific Issues with Crohn's and Exercise

For everyone, but especially for those with Crohn's, it is important not to overtrain. Exercising too much becomes counterproductive. This phenomenon is common among runners. It can also occur among other exercise disciplines. We all know weekend warriors who overdo things after a layoff and hurt or injure themselves, suffering a setback for weeks and months.

There is value to a routine that promotes variety, for example, alternating the type of exercise from walking or running to weight training. Similarly, it makes good sense that if you train hard one day, to take it easy the next day.

People with Crohn's who are seriously exercising will experience more setbacks than those without the disease. The reason is that exercise stresses the body, usually in a good way. But too much physical stress can trigger a Crohn's flare-up or make the body less able to resist other problems such as colds or flu or worse.

The key is to start slow, increase gradually and when you experience a setback, rest and then start again as soon as you are ready. If you are an ex-marine or your former coach taught you to push through an injury, ignore that advice and rest longer than you normally would want to.

Another thing to keep in mind is that as we get older, it takes longer for us to recover, so cultivating patience is recommended. When I'm getting back to exercising after a layoff, a little trick I have learned is to tell myself I am going to exercise 15 minutes, sometimes even just 5 minutes. If I have been slacking off or gotten out of my routine due to fatigue or illness, this makes it easier for me to get started again. After a few days, 15 minutes no longer seems like enough time, at which point I gradually extend my session to 30 or 45 minutes. Generally, 45 minutes is my limit. However, if I am combining my exercise session with yoga or stretching, I will often go 60 minutes or more.

Another thing I have learned over the years—much of it from my study of yoga—is to distinguish "good pain" from "bad pain." The former comes from the burn in the muscles being exercised. The latter is pain felt in any joint, the back, or the neck. When that occurs, it is time to follow the advice in the classic Henny Youngman joke:

> *A man goes to the doctor and says, "Doctor, doctor, it hurts when I do this!" The doctor says, "Don't do this."*

Anytime I have violated this rule, I have paid a big price. A proactive way to deal with pain that occurs while exercising is to find a personal trainer, physical therapist or chiropractor that will work with you. Some of these practitioners are poor, some good, and some are great. As in selecting any health professional, be sure to do your homework. Ask friends for recommendations, check the Internet for reviews, call ahead and ask the office staff questions. Most importantly, if you are not happy with the provider, seek out another.

Nutrition and Exercise

Remember to eat or drink some protein within 30 minutes of exercising. This is important for everyone, but especially for a person with Crohn's. The reason is that the body needs protein in the recovery process.

I like a rice protein added to orange juice and some psyllium husk for fiber. For more protein and some digestive enzymes, I add organic yogurt. This is my "power" drink.

Take

4 ounces of orange juice

4 ounces of water

2 heaping tablespoons of zero or low fat French vanilla organic yogurt

1 serving of rice protein

1/3 to 1/2 serving of smooth or whole husk psyllium fiber

A liquid vitamin and mineral supplement

I mix it in a bottle with a screw-on cap and drink. I use the smooth psyllium husk when my bowels are acting up. Sometimes I double the juice and water, increase the yogurt to 1/4 or 1/2 cup, add a half or whole banana and blend in blender. When I do that, it becomes my breakfast.

Challenges

There are challenges that everyone exercising encounters. Topping the list is boredom. Repetition can be tedious. When the monotony gets to you, change your location or your routine. Cross-training—alternating biking, running and swimming, for example—can help. You may not become a world-class athlete, but you will reduce your chances of repetitive-use injuries and will have a more balanced workout that promotes a more balanced body. Whenever you have more time, go to a park or hiking trail, or to the tennis courts or golf course, for a change of pace.

It is great fun to exercise with a friend, and certainly relieves boredom, but do not depend on it. If your friend is late or sick or loses motivation, your exercise program is sabotaged. I have seen a lot of people use the friend method of working out and the relationships rarely lasted. In fact, I can only remember one that did, and that's because the couple got married. If you need other people around when you exercise, go to the gym. If you can afford it, hire a personal trainer.

Fatigue is another condition that most Crohnies experience. It is certainly one of my biggest challenges all around. I will discuss that in more detail in Chapter 10—Rest, Energy and Sleep.

For now, let's just look at it from an exercise point of view. If your arms or legs feel like they are filled with lead, is it better to push on or just rest? My approach is to walk or bike at whatever pace is comfortable, for about 10 minutes. If the heavy appendages lighten, I pick up the pace or go to my scheduled routine. If they remain heavy, that is it—I'm done for the day—and I give myself permission to rest my body as much as it needs. The next day, I repeat the process. Sometimes it may take days or even weeks to rest and recover. This can be especially discouraging if you had gotten yourself in really good shape. If it is taking weeks to recover, a visit to your doctor may be called for.

Another word of caution: You may have the ability to shine in your age group—certain competitive swimmers, for example, set international records at age 70 and older—but I would think twice before imitating them if you have Crohn's. There are digestive disorders that occur in elite athletes, primarily runners and cyclists, associated with hard training and competing at the marathon or Tour de France levels. They are more common among women than men. In either case, you don't need to do that to yourself. I have run some 5Ks and suffered no problems. Although I've been tempted to train to run a marathon, I don't believe it would be a healthy thing for me. So I just enjoy being in the top 10% of my age group, athletically, and leave the top echelon for others.

Exercise and Habit

A while back, I was having a hard time doing my exercise, so I decided to join a gym. I was doing great until I simply lost my motivation. Yes, I admit to being human and not making the effort to get to the gym. I could say I didn't have the time, but a day always has 24 hours. I only went one day instead of my normal three or four times each week. Then, I was going once every 2 weeks and before I knew it, I was out for a month. I had paid for a year and I wasn't going to throw the money away, so I went back one morning. I happened to see the owner of the gym on the way out and started to talk to him about my difficulties keeping on schedule.

He said, "John, the way to do it is to come down first thing in the morning and get it over with."

I knew he was right.

The key was to have a set time and let nothing stand in my way. The mistake I had made was having a cup of coffee before I went for my workout. I associate coffee with pleasure and a relaxing morning. You might need to have that cup of tea or coffee or whatever before you can get started. If it works for you—great! For me, I had to make it something to look forward to—my coffee as a little reward after my workout. Of course, I had my protein drink first.

So, I returned to going to the gym—no coffee or juice, just water—and was soon back to my five-day, balanced-exercise program. That included 4 days working out, and on one weekend day, either with Colette or by myself, I would go for a bike ride, extended walk or longer run.

Summary

I believe everybody can exercise. I believe everybody must exercise. For exercise to bring one maximum benefit, it has to be a habit, and be done within one's limits. For muscles and bones to be healthy, they must be stressed and rested. Exercise is beneficial and necessary, not only to the bones and muscles, but to all the systems of the body including the brain and the digestive system. Regarding exercise, it is often helpful to remember Mark Twain's quote, 'The secret of getting ahead is getting started."

🌿 *Chapter 7*
YOGA

My sister recently reminded me that I had once told her that yoga saved my life. Maybe what I should have said was that yoga rescued the quality of my life. I began taking classes to improve my flexibility, and being a weekend athlete, to reduce my chances of injury, but over the years, I began to realize that yoga had a positive impact on my life in many other ways. Okay, I admit to being biased—I'm a fan. But there is no doubt in my mind that many of yoga's benefits have played a direct and an indirect role in my ability to successfully manage Crohn's disease.

Although it has become increasingly mainstream—about 20 million people practice it in the United States—many still consider yoga to be exercise for new age types at best. However, the Mayo Clinic, not exactly a new age institution, comments on its website that yoga's health benefits are stress reduction, improved fitness, and chronic disease management.

Other studies have demonstrated that yoga lowers heart rates, blood pressure, blood sugar, cholesterol and atherosclerosis while boosting the immune system and increasing antioxidants in the body. Its ability to improve balance is well known, which is great for everyone and especially seniors because it prevents injury resulting from falls. Not only do people with health problems who practice yoga visit the hospital less frequently, but they also need fewer drugs.

It is no wonder, then, that yoga has been, for some years, a resource for scientists and a few practitioners in the medical community looking for ways to supplement conventional methods. One of the more widely known is *The Spectrum*—a program created by Dean Ornish, M.D. for heart patients, which includes yoga as a part of the treatment along with diet and other low cost, but effective, techniques. Ornish, a physician and clinical professor of medicine, developed his approach as a preventative, more lifestyle-driven alternative to surgery and drug treatments of coronary artery disease and other chronic ailments. In the beginning, although successful, his discoveries were considered only for the highly motivated and highly disciplined. Today, the Dean Ornish program is paid for by many insurance companies as well as by Medicare.

Yoga differs from regular exercise. Generally, it is a slow-moving activity involving static postures, fluid motion, and low impact activities. On the other hand, conventional exercise usually involves faster movement and forceful repetitions. Yoga places much more emphasis on controlling the breath and awareness of body position. More advanced yoga focuses on subtle energy flow and draws the attention inward.

As William J. Broad points out in his book, *The Science of Yoga,* there are health benefits for the average, as well as the advanced yoga practitioner.

Yoga and Crohn's Disease

Perhaps the most important benefit for those with Crohn's is yoga's ability to diminish stress. It has also been found that stress reduction boosts immunity and prevents disease. This is one reason why clinical studies indicate patients who do yoga go to the hospital less often and need less medicine.

Another great benefit of yoga for Crohnies is that it encourages them to exercise more control of the nervous system. That, in turn, leads to stimulating the part of the nervous system that regulates the immune system and the digestive system.

How does yoga have that kind of impact? The nervous system functions in two different modes, voluntary and involuntary. We have conscious control over the former—we think about moving an arm or leg muscle before we do it, even if it is only a fraction of a second. The latter happens without our conscious input—we don't think about engaging the heart and digestive system muscles for them to do their jobs.

The operation of the involuntary, or autonomic system, can be broken down into two subcategories—the sympathetic and the parasympathetic system. The sympathetic system mobilizes the body for activities such as stimulating the adrenal gland. The parasympathetic system conserves energy and promotes housekeeping functions such as digesting our food during rest. Obviously, we need both of these systems.

Problems occur when these two systems are out of whack. This is especially true if one has a chronic health problem such as Crohn's disease. Scientific studies, as well as my own experience, indicate that practicing yoga helps keep these two essential systems in equilibrium and can aid in restoring their proper balance.

Other Benefits

Another benefit for people with Crohn's is the ability to develop healthier posture through yoga. Proper posture leads to good spinal alignment, which in turn is good for the nervous, pulmonary and circulatory systems, not to mention the skeletal and muscular systems. Did I mention the digestive system? Yes, that too. Yoga creates openness in the body which promotes good health. Your intestines can actually stick together. The postures of yoga can promote the gut aligning itself optimally. Above all, good posture can lead to a better attitude; if you stand, sit and move well, it is bound to affect how you feel about yourself and life in general. By the way, my posture at 68 is much better than it was before I discovered yoga 28 years ago.

The process of doing the yoga postures also flushes out toxins and brings in fresh oxygen via blood. The body produces, takes in, and stores toxins. Obviously, we want to get rid of them as soon as we can. Exercise creates toxins and gets rid of them. Yoga postures actually act like a massage for your organs. You bend forward, backward, and to the sides, and twist to the right and left in a way you normally wouldn't, stimulating muscle cells and acting as a release and cleanse.

The twisting and flexing of the spine during yoga practice gets blood to the intervertebral discs. This is a very good thing because these discs, although essential to posture and everything that involves the backbone, do not have their own blood vessels. When human life spans were shorter, that didn't matter. However, in the 21st century, we live longer and are only as old, or young, as our spine.

When I was doing yoga teacher training, about every month or two there would be a special class dedicated to opening the hips. These classes were more intense than what you would get in a normal class or workshop. For 2 or 3 days afterward, I would be extremely fatigued. After taking several of these classes, I just expected I would not have much energy for a few days. Well, after a year or more, I was fine—no fatigue. What was the difference? I believe I was releasing toxins that were stored in my body, perhaps from my surgeries or having been around pesticides, or what not, but I feel strongly that I got rid of some bad stuff that was stored in my hip and gut area.

Yoga and Emotions

Yet another benefit of the practice of yoga is that it can lift one's mood. This seems to benefit women more than men. According to a study by the National Center for Health Statistics, women are 2 ½ times more likely to be on antidepressants than men. When I attended and taught yoga classes, women always outnumbered men by a wide margin, and I thought it was because they enjoyed the non-competitive, low impact type of activity. As a rule, women are more flexible than men, so it was something they excelled in and could enjoy. Perhaps that had something to do with it, but now I also think that maybe it was because women received something they needed on a deeper psychological level.

Scientists have found that even for beginning students, not just more advanced yogis, practicing yoga increases a chemical in the brain—gamma-amino-butyric acid or GABA for short—that plays a major role in preventing depression. For years, I heard from women in my yoga classes that they loved going to weekend yoga workshops. I thought it was just a woman thing and it made no sense to me. They cost too much and took up too much time. However, after a painful divorce, I grew to love and look forward to those workshops myself. I thought they were something to do to fill my time and hone my skills. Little did I know that they may have met a more basic need. I was getting my GABA levels lifted and didn't even know it.

Does the increase in GABA levels have anything to do with Crohn's management? Studies show that one's mental state reduces the intensity of disease and aids in the healing process. I believe that a person with Crohn's who is in a good mood most of the time has a better life than someone with no health problems who is in a perpetually bad mood.

Yoga and Breath

Breath is life. We can survive for days without water and weeks without food, but will not last much longer than 5 minutes without air. Okay, so you know how to breathe—it's part of the body's involuntary systems. Yet, yoga can teach you how to do it more efficiently.

Most of us take breaths that are too shallow. I was once taught that we should breathe from the stomach and for years, when I wanted to "do it correctly," I used my stomach muscles. Wrong! When breathing, the stomach muscles should be relaxed and the stomach will rise and fall on its own because the diaphragm pushes down as it expands the lungs without any help from the stomach muscles.

I believe learning to relax my stomach muscles was an important factor in becoming more successful at managing my Crohn's. Like many other Americans, I was unconsciously contracting my stomach muscles. The digestive tract does not function optimally surrounded by chronically tight stomach muscles.

The husband of one of my regular yoga students joined my class for the first time after he and his wife returned from a winter spent in the Caribbean. They were an adventurous couple who lived in a tent campground when on the islands and he made his living there as a scuba diving instructor. When they came home, he worked as a home building contractor and she created sculptures. He had never attended a yoga class, and I was surprised to see him. After class, he explained it baffled him that his wife, for the first time, was able to stay underwater longer than him. At some point, they put two and two together and realized the reason: after a year in my yoga classes, she had learned how to breathe more efficiently and to control her breath even when in a stressful, yet exciting situation, like scuba diving. I had a motivated, new yoga student, and soon he learned to breathe more efficiently, too.

Knowing how to control one's breath is also a great tool when dealing with any negative or stressful situation. I use it at the dentist's office and before giving a speech, as well as when my digestion is challenged due to worry or tension.

Medical science has begun to realize the importance of breath and health. An article titled "Inflammation: nutritional, botanical and mind-body influences," written by two physicians (D.P. Rakel & A. Rindfleisch) appeared in the March 2005 edition of the Southern Medical Journal and pointed out the value of doing certain simple breathing exercises. Apparently, this kind of breath work stimulates the vagus nerve, the longest in the body, whose function includes regulating the heartbeat, informing the brain when food is ingested and digested, and emptying the gastric region of waste material.

It also prevents the release of the Tumor Necrosis Factor (TNF), which triggers an inflammatory response, a cause of many problems of autoimmune disorders, including Crohn's. There are drugs to combat the inflammatory response. But unlike TNF drugs, doing breathwork, to my knowledge, has no dangerous side effects. While some patients may require TNF drugs to reduce the inflammatory response, I interpret these findings to mean that others can use simple breathing exercises on a daily basis instead, along with the other practices described in this book.

Yoga and Crohn's

One of the most important benefits yoga offers to any chronic illness like Crohn's is its emphasis on awareness and release of tension. A National Institution of Health publication titled "Crohn's disease—discharge" recommends reducing muscle tension and that one way to learn it is through yoga.

In the style of yoga I studied, awareness is taught beginning with the shape of the postures. This relates to awareness of everyday posture, and posture is very important to breathing and digestion. As soon as students begin to learn the shape of a pose, they are encouraged to be aware of muscle tension throughout the body. Once they are alert to posture and muscle tightness, they can begin to focus on their breathing. Tension and stress affect breath, making it more rapid, shorter, and more shallow. Conversely, tension and stress can be reduced by slowing, lengthening and deepening the breath. This is an extremely valuable tool for a Crohn's patient who wants to reduce stress. It's impossible to modify one's breath and to create healthier breathing habits without being first aware. I had little to no awareness of my breath, muscle tension, or even my posture before I practiced yoga.

Balance

Another benefit of practicing yoga is attaining good balance. The advantages of a better equilibrium may not be as obvious for Crohn's patients as those of awareness. But it is just as important. Health and yoga are very much about finding balance, for example, the balance between work and rest. A good yoga class is neither all about effort nor all about relaxation. Contrast this with other exercise classes. Most of them are all about effort.

It is important for everyone to have balance in their lives but especially for Crohn's patients. If a 100% healthy individual works too hard or eats an unbalanced diet, it will show up much later than if a Crohn's patient does the same. To the outsider or the beginner, it looks as if yoga balance is about standing on one foot, but the real balance taught in a good yoga class is about finding equanimity in that class and eventually bringing that practice into everyday life.

In my own life, I had to learn it was okay to not work so hard. I believe this translates to any path a Crohnie may choose. An accountant with Crohn's may have to give up the thrill and extra stress of tax season. A truck driver may have to find local instead of the long distance runs he loves because of the limited food choices available at truck-stops. Everyone must find his or her own point of equilibrium. The balance point is just a little finer for someone challenged by Crohn's.

My Yoga Journey

I first went to yoga classes with some notion that I needed to stretch my muscles. I was not a great student. I never read a book on yoga. I didn't want the teacher to touch me. I tried too hard to get in positions I couldn't do, in spite of the instructor telling us to stay within our limits. It was years before I practiced outside of class and even then, I did the bare minimum. In retrospect, it seems amazing that I kept going to classes once a week. It may have had something to do with luck and the fact that my first teacher was a certified Iyengar instructor, well-trained and impressive. In fact, all of my teachers have had their initial training in this type of yoga.

B.K.S. Iyengar, the man who developed the yoga that is named for him, is a native of India. He is over 90 years old and still practices his yoga which focuses on healthy alignment of the musculoskeletal system with more emphasis on the physical rather than the spiritual aspect. Iyengar was mentored by an Indian surgeon earlier in his career and developed an understanding of the anatomy of the human body that is unique among yoga teachers, allowing his students to go deeper into postures and get greater muscle stretch.

Realizing that I needed to stretch my muscles may have been the reason I started yoga. Crohn's disease was why I stayed with it. Then the divorce from my wife of 15 years, which caught me by surprise, made me dive in hook, line and sinker. I bought video tapes, attended the weekend workshop, which earlier had seemed like a waste of time and money to me, and practiced more outside of class. I started traveling 40 miles every Saturday morning to atttend a Vinyasa class. It was both more physically challenging and at the same time, more meditative than the one in my hometown.

For me, the best way to learn something really well is to teach it, so I signed up and was accepted to the Iyengar Yoga Institute of San Francisco, a two-year teacher training program. While in California, I also attended Rodney Yee's one-year, yoga teacher training course. Rodney Yee is the yogi in the Pranasleep® mattress ads on television, and he has made lots of yoga videos that are sold in stores, besides being an excellent instructor. In addition, I took numerous other yoga classes and workshops. To say that yoga was the center of my life from September of 1996 until June of 1998 would be a gross understatement. In the course of those 2 years, I probably had more yoga training than 99% of yoga teachers today. I returned to my hometown, started up the Yoga Studio of Murfreesboro, and taught 8 to 10 classes of yoga a week for 7 years.

Getting into Yoga

Based on my many years of training and practice, here is my suggestion for getting going. As with exercise, start gradually and pay attention to your body.

If you do not look out for your own safety and welfare, you may be at risk. This is true in anything you do. A friend who had ridden motorcycles for years attended the beginner class to support his wife, who was a true beginner. Because of his experience, he was assigned a little motor scooter more beat up than the others. When the instructor challenged him to stop in less time than the others, the bent fender on his bike caught the wheel and flipped him, causing him a serious leg injury. He told me later that he had had a bad feeling about what he was being asked to do, but did it anyway. He knows that he should have listened to his intuition. The same holds true in a yoga class. If you have a bad feeling about something, whether beginner or advanced, do not do it.

Once you have researched the classes in your area, talk to the teacher and find out how much training and experience he or she has. Remember, a certification doesn't necessarily mean anything more than the paper it is printed on. Some yoga teachers are very charismatic and exude confidence in their beliefs. Many, like all human beings, are imperfect. Ask other students what they like about the teacher and the classes.

You should ask the teachers what the policy is on touching their students and how much force they use if they do. It might be prudent to ask them to refrain from touching you in the beginning. Some teachers understand the body and how they can assist a student getting into a posture. Many, in my opinion, do not.

Once you decide, just pay for one class, not a series, even though it is more expensive per class, so you can experience the teacher firsthand and decide if you wish to continue.

A Small Yoga Library

I recommended the following yoga books to my students:

How to Use Yoga by Mira Mehta. This book is great for beginners. The explanation and pictures of the postures are excellent. A 10-week course with a daily 30 minute practice, it has small pictures of the postures so the practice is not constantly broken up, flipping back to see what the posture should look like. In addition, the pictures and names of the postures are referenced so that they are easy to find if more detailed instruction is desired.

Back Care Basics: a Doctor's Gentle Yoga Program for Back and Neck Pain Relief by Mary Pullig Schatz, M.D., with a preface by B.K.S. Iyenger, is for anyone that needs to tread lightly with their yoga practice. It is good for anyone that is a bit stiff due to age, injury or whatever, as well as those suffering from back and neck issues.

Yoga: The Iyengar Way by Silva, Mira, and Shyam Mehta is an advanced book for those that want to take their yoga practice to a higher level.

The Science of Yoga: The Risks and the Rewards by William J. Broad, is not an instruction book. The author is a Pulitzer Prize-winning journalist who has practiced yoga since 1970. This is a well-researched book that covers all aspects of the practice. It includes the history of yoga and explains in layman's terms the scientific research of yoga's many benefits. It also details what goes on in modern yoga classes, covering the good, the bad, and what to be cautious about regarding postures and teachers.

There are many good yoga DVDs out there. Start with the beginner ones and work up. I prefer the Iyengar instructional DVDs.

When considering the cost of classes, DVDs are inexpensive, since they can be used over and over.

Books and DVDs are great but nothing is as great as a good teacher. In addition, the energy we all get from being in a class with others keeps us going.

❧ *Chapter 8*
MEDITATION

Meditation is often thought of in connection with new-age, spiritual quests or eastern religious traditions, in which practitioners chant obscure "mantras" silently in their heads. However, meditation does not have to be connected to either to be used as a tool for better health. Scientific studies have shown that meditation can reduce chronic pain, anxiety, high blood pressure, cholesterol levels, and drug abuse. It can slow the heart rate, increase blood flow, and promote a relaxed but alert state. Obviously, all these things could be helpful to anyone challenged with Crohn's disease.

Meditation is different from prayer. It is not in competition with it. In fact, neuroscientific studies conducted by Dr. Andrew Newberg, MD, of Thomas Jefferson University Hospital and Medical College, found that a different part of the brain is engaged for prayer than for meditation. In prayer, the frontal lobe, the language and the focusing areas of the brain, comes into play just as in a normal conversation. Meditation utilizes none of these areas. To put it into simple terms, the brain is relaxed in meditation and engaged in prayer. This, as well as my own experience with prayer and meditation, has led me to believe that if the goal is to reduce stress, meditation is important whether one engages in prayer or not.

I discovered meditation in 1995 when I was going through my divorce and felt stressed, agitated, and unhappy much of the time. In a bookstore, I stumbled upon *Zen Keys* by Thich Nhat Hanh. For some reason, the philosophy made sense to me, so I bought another of Hanh's books, *The Miracle of Mindfulness: An Introduction to the Practice of Meditation*, and put his suggestions into practice. Soon after, I started to meditate 15 to 30 minutes a day. Before long, I felt a sense of peace I hadn't in some time, and while I wasn't happy about my divorce, I was getting closer to accepting it.

I consider meditation to be very important in my management of Crohn's. A major benefit is that when I am less tense and more relaxed, my digestive tract functions better and my Crohn's is less active. Because I am more mindful, I pay closer attention to my diet and eat more of the "good" foods I need and eat less of the "bad" foods I want. I am also more focused and get more work done while expending less energy. In addition, my exercise regime and yoga practice are more consistent, paying additional health dividends.

There have been unexpected gains as well. Not only does meditation aid in my ability to concentrate, it has allowed me to become less judgmental. Surprisingly, I have found that it helps me forgive others and myself more quickly. And indirectly, it has had positive effects on my posture and breath.

One of the great things about meditation is that it can be done by anyone just about anywhere, without having to buy any equipment, and with little instruction. All that is needed is a floor and cushion or a chair. It is also easy to restart if you have taken a break from it. Sit for five or 10 minutes the first day and add 5 minutes every day or two after that, and before long, you will be meditating as long as you want.

Even though an aspect of meditation is to be alert, do not meditate while driving or doing anything that has the potential to be dangerous, if you're not paying full attention.

How to Meditate

I sit on a cushion or chair. The cushion can be a folded blanket. If I'm on the floor, I sit with my legs crossed. I have experimented and found the positions that work best for me. If you are not a yogi, I recommend a chair with a firm, cushioned seat. Do not make contact with the back of the chair.

First, I focus on my grounding. If I am on a cushion on the floor, I make sure my sitting bones—the ischial tuberosity of the pelvis—are firmly and evenly making contact with the cushion or blanket. Next, I make sure my knees are touching the blanket or mat. It is important to have the knees grounded so use a blanket or books to give them the support they need to rest comfortably. If I am sitting on a chair, I sit with my sitting bones evenly on the seat, my two feet on the floor. The heels are under my knees, which are about hip width (the width of the sitting bones) apart. There are other ways to sit for meditation but either variation works for me, and one or both will work for you, too.

Once my grounding is established, I focus on my posture. I lift up through the spine, draw my shoulders slightly back and make sure my lower back has its natural curve. I relax my shoulders. Then I lift the center of my head toward the ceiling and ever so slightly, tilt the chin down. My legs, torso, head and neck are positioned. I let my hands rest on my thighs, palms up or down. Sometimes, I softy interlock my fingers and with the thumbs on the upside, I bring the tips of the thumbs together. There are other ways to hold the hands; all of them are the "right" way.

Once I have established the posture of my body, I concentrate on my muscles making sure that my legs, hips, and belly muscles are completely relaxed. The muscles that keep my back, neck, head, arms and hands in place are engaged, but not rigid. I also relax the throat and facial muscles. When beginning the practice, especially if I am starting back after some time off, I often make a muscle group rigid and then relax them to the desired amount of toning. I might do each group two or three times to get my muscles just the way I want them, and to imprint in my brain as well as the muscles the state I want them in. I even check the eye muscles, "softening" the eyes by looking slightly downward.

I like to keep my eyes open and slightly unfocused. Other forms of meditation encourage closed eyes. Either works. Remember, there is no such thing as a right or wrong way to meditate, although with eyes closed, it's easier to go to sleep, which defeats the purpose of meditation.

Then I begin to observe the breath. It is important to not try to change it during a meditation practice, but to work on it at another time. The breath is connected to the posture and the muscles. If I am slumping, it makes my breathing more shallow. If I pull my shoulders back too far, the breath will be affected. If I am holding my belly muscles or my neck muscles, the breath will not flow as it should. It is said one cannot observe the breath without changing the breath, so I concentrate on making the conditions right for a smooth, even breath, while forgiving myself when I realize I am not letting the breath be natural.

This preparation will take from 1 to 5 minutes, depending on how regularly I have meditated. When I first started, it took longer. I am now ready to begin meditating. The idea is to focus the mind on one thing. This can be an object, a candle, a word, a phrase, a mantra, counting to 10 over and over. What one chooses to concentrate on may or may not provide additional benefits. However, the most important benefit is that it keeps the mind from drifting, from being a busy mind. Again, this differs from prayer, which may focus on many things. This is why both prayer and meditation can be beneficial to a Crohn's patient, and why one does not need to exclude the other.

I frequently find that all kinds of thoughts and images intrude—recent experiences, distant memories, things I worry about, or am trying to solve. When that happens, I take notice and bring myself to focus on what I have decided to meditate on for that session.

When my meditation is steady, I sit for 30 minutes a day. For a long time, I did 15-minute meditations. I have gone for as little as 5 minutes, but find I don't experience much benefit until I make it at least a quarter of an hour. Still, I believe 5 minutes is better than no meditation. Some people sit for longer, up to 2 hours a day. There may be periods in one's life where such extended meditation might be helpful, during times of great turmoil like divorce, illness, or death of a loved one. In normal circumstances, I believe it could be harmful and may be more of an escape mechanism than a tool for a better life. But that is just my opinion.

I use a simple timer with a soft ping. Sometimes, I start thinking about the time about 5 minutes before the timer goes off. At other times, there is the mind game that occurs when the question "Did I set the timer?" enters my thoughts. Looking at the timer in the middle of a meditation spoils the effect, so to avoid doing so I have learned to set the timer, punch start, put it down and then pick it up again, look at it and consciously say to myself, "It is counting down," before starting.

Another important aspect is to approach meditation in a nonjudgmental way. If I find myself forgetting what I am focusing on, I simply go back to focusing on that word, or object, or whatever. When I realize I am slumping, I go back to a more erect, but natural posture. When I realize my breath is more shallow than normal, I check my muscles, especially my belly muscles. I even check my thoughts. Have I allowed anger, judgment or worry to seep in? Anything that doesn't belong to what I am trying to practice is subject to correction. It's not only okay to "mess-up" during meditation, it's regarded as part of the process. What is not acceptable is to quit because we make mistakes or don't forgive ourselves for our "mess-ups."

Like all of the things I do to mitigate my Crohn's disease, sometimes I neglect meditation and have to get back on track. At times like that, I become more aware of its many benefits. After a period of no meditation, and then having a regular meditation practice for about a month, meditation seems more natural, and its benefits: relaxation, stress reduction, better digestion, more focus, better discipline, being less judgmental and more mindful, to name a few, start to multiply.

Meditation and Yoga

There is no substitute for sitting meditation. However, there are ways to enhance activities by practicing meditation in action. It can be done while at the gym, when cleaning the floor, during gardening, even while preparing a meal. Some describe this state as being "in the zone" with a greater focus and awareness of what they are doing.

The type of yoga I studied emphasizes the physical. The founder, B.K.S. Iyengar likes to say that the physical practice of yoga is meditation in action. What I believe he was saying is that one can do yoga and go in and out of the postures in such a way that they are meditative.

Let me take this notion a step further. Let's say you go to the gym. Rock and Roll music is blaring from speakers and from time to time someone interrupts, saying hi or engaging in conversation with you. Is it possible, then, to make it a meditation or a yoga practice despite external intrusions? I think so. It's not that difficult once you get the hang of it.

If you are working out with weights, make sure you don't use more than you can lift with good form. Soften your eyes by looking slightly downward and focus on your breath and posture, just as you would in a sitting meditation practice. As you lift the weights, continue to focus on them as well as your form while lifting the weights. As you move from one exercise station to another, concentrate on walking with mindfulness and awareness. If someone says hi, smile and return the greeting. If someone engages you in conversation, then you are no longer meditating, but as soon as you're done, go back to making your workout a meditation.

When I taught yoga, very few of my students got this. They had set in their mind that meditation required sitting still. I wish I had been a better teacher. I think I was able to learn that a workout could be a meditation because I had the advantage of having years of practicing yoga and a two-year period when I studied it full time.

Further Reading

There are numerous books on both the theory and practice of meditation.

If you prefer a more spiritual approach, I would recommend the earlier-mentioned *The Miracle of Mindfulness: An Introduction to the Practice of Meditation* by Thich Nhat Hanh, one of the best known and most respected Zen masters in the world today, a poet, and a peace and human rights activist.

If you prefer a more basic, beginner's approach, consider *Meditation For Dummies* by Stephan Bodian, a meditation teacher and licensed psychotherapist with an expertise in stress management. (I have only read the mini-edition, Kindle version.)

For something in between, *Feel Better Now…Meditation for Stress Reduction and Relaxation* by Gary Halperin is a simple straightforward explanation of meditation written by a certified professional level Kripalu Yoga teacher and meditation teacher.

Summary

By practicing sitting meditation, we can learn to use some or all of its techniques in any part of our life, from going to a busy mall to attending an emotional funeral. One caution, though, to beginners taking meditation into the world: It does not mean going out in a dreamy state. It means being totally alert, with energy appropriate for whatever task or behavior you are doing.

I won't claim that meditation or any other single practice has been the most important factor in living well with Crohn's, but I can say that for me, it has been a very important part of the foundation.

❧ *Chapter 9*
STRESS MANAGEMENT

Every stress leaves an indelible scar, and the organism
pays for its survival after a stressful situation
by becoming a little older.
—Hans Selye

In 1920, Hans Selye, a Hungarian endocrinologist whom many consider the father of stress research, conducted studies that led him to believe that stress had biological roots. He developed a theory that stress was a general strain on the body caused by atypical body functions which then caused a release in hormones. He called this the General Adaptation Syndrome or our body's long or short term response to stress. Selye was certain that stress impacted health. Not all of his colleagues agreed.

In time, other researchers verified his findings and discovered more physiological, as well as psychological, triggers. In one study, a group of unfed monkeys not watching neighbors eat had much lower levels of stress hormones than the unfed group watching their neighbors feasting on tasty bananas and oranges. Research became more specific over time, but it was more and more understood that both physical and mental stress can affect health adversely.

Yet even today, almost 100 years later, many medical practitioners, including some gastroenterologists, don't believe in the importance of managing stress for better health, even though their denial flies in the face of increasing documentation in professional journals linking stress and illness.

- As early as 1986, the Journal of Advanced Nursing reported on a one-year study of patients with inflammatory bowel disease (IBD). The results suggested that stress management techniques may have therapeutic benefits for IBD patients.

- A 1991 report in the Journal of Behavioral Medicine concluded that for some individuals with Crohn's disease, daily stress is related to their confirming symptoms which indicated they had the illness.

- A 2004 report in the American Journal of Gastroenterology found that psychological distress was associated with the cause and development of functional GI disorders.

- Another 2004 report, published in Behavior Research and Therapy and titled "A stress management programme for Crohn's disease" determined that the patients who received training in self-directed stress management techniques experienced reductions in tiredness and abdominal pain.

It has been estimated that two-thirds of all doctor visits are at least partially related to stress. The Mayo Clinic listed 125 stress-related illnesses. The 10 top listed on WebMD (www.webmd.com) are heart disease, asthma, obesity, diabetes, headaches, depression and anxiety, gastrointestinal problems, Alzheimer's disease, accelerated aging and premature death. Need I say more?

My Own History

My original gastroenterologist, a hard-charging kind of guy, liked to point out that stress was part of life. One time, probably speaking from personal experience, he mentioned that making money equaled stress. While both statements are undoubtedly true, he had no good answers for what to do about it other than to live with it. However, 20 or so years later, he began to realize that managing stress was important and tried to find ways to make it part of his practice—both for himself and for his patients. My hat is off to him for being willing to learn and grow.

Thinking back on how and when I learned to manage stress, I muddled along until, due to want or necessity, I eventually changed my direction. When I was first diagnosed with Crohn's, I made no adjustments. After three hospital visits over the course of a few months, I decided to slow down a bit. While going through my second divorce, I really learned about managing stress. The tools were right in front of my eyes, but it took a divorce before I could see them. It was doing yoga, along with the biofeedback techniques I was learning from yoga, that taught me the most about stress management.

However, not everyone will have the opportunity or desire to practice yoga, so this chapter is about many of the other available stress management techniques. Some of these tools were pioneered by yogis and later refined and westernized by modern scientists. Most have nothing to do with yoga.

Before we go any further, let's not disparage stress. Like many things that have a bad reputation, on reflection, we realize stress can be good or it can be bad. Stress promotes creativity. A comfortable mind has no reason to see things differently. Stress aids in problem solving. A person who doesn't care, will not worry and will not have reason to deal with harmful emotions or situations. Stress enhances physical performance because it speeds up heart rate and metabolism, thus improving reflexes and even acting as a pain killer. Stress on muscles is essential to build strength and endurance.

There is one thing that all of the above and any other positive-stress factors have in common. Too much and/or too prolonged stress turns negative. Therefore, the challenge is how to harness and control our stress.

Stress and Biology

When our car won't start on our child's first day in school, or we owe an extra $10,000 to the IRS that we don't have, or we suffer from a bad toothache, the body experiences stress and responds by releasing the stress hormones adrenaline and cortisol. Adrenaline has an electrochemical nature and is a neurotransmitter that carries nerve impulses to target cells. Adrenaline levels surge when the body perceives threats, what is commonly known as the "fight-or-flight" response. This psychological reaction has its root in prehistoric times when our ancestors dealt with direct threats by either standing their ground and putting up a fight, or running away. Heart rate and blood pressure increase. As blood vessels contract, the air passages expand. We feel energized, more alert and ready to tackle life's challenges.

The other stress hormone, cortisol, is a natural corticosteroid released gradually by the adrenal glands. Cortisol helps rid the body of toxins and improves short term memory, and most important for Crohn's patients, reduces inflammation. On the surface, that would seem to be a good thing. But it seems that chronic stress, which leads to prolonged secretion of these hormones, limits their effectiveness over time, causing white blood cells, for example, to lose their ability to respond to anti-inflammatory signals.

The above studies, as well as my personal experience, strongly suggest that both past and present stress may contribute to Crohn's disease and health in general. It has made sense to me for some time to strive to manage stressors and their effects to the best of my ability, and I have gladly reaped the rewards of greater joy and happiness all around.

Stress Management Tools

WebMD lists the following ways to relieve stress:

- writing
- letting out your feelings (talking, crying, laughing, etc.)

- doing something you enjoy (hobbies, volunteering, sports)
- focusing on the present
- exercising regularly
- meditating
- breathing exercises
- practicing yoga, tai chi and qigong

Writing

I am not talking about becoming an author. The process of writing and publishing a book has plenty of stressful times. Some have likened it metaphorically to giving birth. For me, it has been more like a job. Some of it is fun, but there are factors that make it stressful, notably being a novice at the writing game and starting out knowing nothing about the process or what it takes to publish and promote a book.

There have been times in my life, however, when writing for myself brought me considerable relief from pressure, tension and constant worry. During one period when I was trying to accomplish so much with so little, I would wake up at night, and toss and turn for hours, thinking of all the things I had to accomplish the next day. I found that putting a pad and pen on the nightstand by the bed helped a great deal. If I turned on the light and wrote down the ideas or plans, I could let go of what I was brooding about, clear my mind, and go back to sleep.

I have known individuals who considered daily journaling essential to their mental health. They often have a set time when they put down thoughts, feelings, and events that occurred that day. The key, I believe, is not to worry about how it comes out or whether grammar and spelling are correct. Just let it flow onto the page or iPad.

Letting out your feelings

I was recently at a funeral of a 67-year-old man, a co-worker of Colette's, who had died in a motorcycle accident a few months before he was going to retire. The chapel was full, standing room only. All of the speakers, except for the man's supervisor and friend, were members of an Alcoholics Anonymous organization. I had never been at a funeral where so many men spoke so freely. Their love and respect for their dead friend was amazing. Although dressed in their best dark suits, some of them were a little rough around the edges. It was impressive to see a group of men, who were more macho than touchy-feely, get up and share their feelings so openly, laughing and crying comfortably in public. I understand this is one of the steps AA recommends in combating alcoholism. Still, these guys were exemplary.

I'll admit that expressing my feelings doesn't come easy to me and I have had to work on it. I guess I'm rather stoic by nature. I used to feel that I shouldn't burden others by talking about my Crohn's disease. I was fine speaking to a group or talking and joking with friends. I could even cry at movies, usually when I was alone. However, when it came to talking about my own feelings, I would clam up. It has taken time and the encouragement of others, notably my wife, for me to share my emotions. I also think my yoga training has helped to open me up, so that I can talk about most things affecting me now. That does not mean I go around jabbering at length about my feelings or health problems. When conversation turns to Crohn's, I keep it brief and upbeat. If people want to know more, I will gladly share more about myself from a positive, but realistic perspective.

If you are someone who has difficulty with letting your emotions out, there are lots of ways to get there. For some, it might mean joining a group like the AA mentioned above. There is actually a 12 step program called Emotions Anonymous. For others, it might take counseling or therapy. For those less challenged, perhaps joining Toastmasters and just talking will do the trick. Any of these will probably release some stress hormones, and over time may relax the need for others.

Doing something you enjoy

We all know people so driven to succeed that they work at all hours and never take the time to "smell the roses," as the saying goes. But what is the use of life if you can't enjoy it? Maybe because my childhood was more focused on work than play—growing up on a farm, I had to do a lot of daily chores—I decided at some point that I was going to set aside some time for what I enjoyed.

In college, I began to learn about leisure activities as well as my studies. Even though I had a job in addition to carrying a full class load, I made time for intramural football, judo, tennis (at a beginner's level) and my all-time favorite pastime, skydiving. The adrenalin rush of falling 120 to 180 miles an hour for 2 miles and then floating gently to the ground was amazing, and I didn't mind dealing with comments like, "Only a fool would jump out of an airplane voluntarily."

Graduation, marriage and Vietnam ended my skydiving adventures, but I found other pastimes, including canoeing and camping with my wife and children (and our dog). After going through my first divorce, I decided to learn how to really play tennis. I actually found standing on painted asphalt in the bright Florida sun and repeatedly hitting a soft little yellow ball back to a person or machine, a lot of fun, and it had a calming effect on my adrenal neurotransmitters.

I also enjoyed volunteering with the Boy Scouts and coaching little league baseball.

I realize that most of my hobbies are physical and sports or nature related. For others it may be reading for pleasure, building models, painting, and many other activities. I know a fellow Crohnie who has an elaborate model train set in his garage where he spends hours and hours building, creating and conducting. If what you do calms and relaxes you, it's probably a good thing.

Because things inevitably change in life, it is a good idea to develop more than one hobby or interest. When my elbow and knee said "no mas" to tennis, I focused on yoga and kayaking, and subsequently on sailing. Probably my favorite stress reliever now is cruising around the outer islands of the Everglades National Park for a week in a small sailboat with my wife. It really calms the body and spirit. Should my body let me down completely, I'll still have chess. I am not very good, but I love the game. If my mind lets me down, well, at that point, all bets are off.

Although I know a lot of guys that have a hard time finding something they enjoy doing, I think more women have this problem. I know some very smart and accomplished women. A much smaller percentage of them than their husbands have pastimes that give them pleasure. It may be because they are so other-directed, always doing things for their families and friends in addition to their busy jobs, that they've never figured out how to take time for themselves.

One exception I know of is the volunteers at my wife's office— her job is volunteer coordinator for a large organization—who are spending part of their retirement "giving back." What sets these retirees apart from their counterparts is that they almost always have a spring in their step, a sparkle in their eye, and something positive to say. Want to reduce stress? Help someone else.

For a long time I believed that watching TV, playing video games and shopping were not stress relievers. However, after more study and thought, I believe they can be, if used in moderation.

One caution: There is a popular saying, mostly among younger men and women, "Work hard, play hard." My feeling is, that approach creates more stress, rather than offer relief from it, and for those with Crohn's, it is downright counterproductive. The point of engaging in a pleasurable hobby or activity is to relax, not get wound up even tighter.

Focusing on the present

In the 1960s, Ram Dass coined the phrase, "Be here now," meaning to be present rather than dwelling on the past or future. When people are asked why they climb Mount Everest, they often answer, "Because I am totally focused on the present, and it makes me feel alive." That seems like an extreme, dangerous, and non recommended way to achieve what I can experience on a good day of warm water sailing or in a good 15-minute meditation, yet I respect those who mountain climb, whether they're aiming their sights for the tallest or some lesser peak.

When I look to the past, I tend to think about what I could have done better. Looking to the future, I tend to think about all the obstacles I must overcome to get to where I am going. Both are stressful. I realize that some of that is due to my bad mental habits, and I know people who can get good feelings from certain memories or by imagining themselves doing something outstanding or exciting down the road. One of my relatives likes to set travel dates to some special place, more than a year ahead of time, so she and her family have something to look forward to.

However, the friends who receive my award for best living in the present, while cultivating a good sense of adventure, are a 40-something couple who have limited time off and a modest travel budget. On the first day of their annual vacation, one of them blindly places a finger on a map, and that is where they go. There are always big smiles on their faces when they describe a past trip or anticipate a future one.

Being in nature

In my case, it's almost as easy as walking out my back door. Like many communities in Florida, mine has nature preserves and walking trails close by. For others, especially city dwellers, it may be more challenging. For them, I recommend spending part of the day on the porch, balcony, or in the back yard and having a meal, solving a puzzle, pursuing a hobby, or doing the daily meditation or exercise.

Or go to the nearest park. If you are shy like me and don't want to do your yoga or resistance exercises in public, just go for a walk, run or bike ride there. Remember, the people you meet are there for the same reason as you, so you don't have to worry about what they are thinking. Early mornings are my favorite time, but any time you can go is great. On the weekends, consider taking a drive to a park further away that offers a different nature experience.

Develop a hobby that gets you out of doors. Fishing, canoeing, kayaking, paddle boarding and sailing are great if you like the water. They can be inexpensive or moderately expensive. Of course, sailing can cost a pretty penny. However, there is a saying among small boaters that the smaller the boat, the more it is used. When we moved to Florida, I planned on buying a 35-foot, used sailboat, which was in my budget. However, I decided to get a 21-footer first because I wanted to hone my skills and learn about which vessel would be best for the local waters before graduating to my dream boat. To make a long story short, I still have a 21-foot boat, different from the one I initially purchased, and more suited to what my wife and I like to do.

Other hobbies that can get you into nature include hiking, bird watching, hunting and photography. Camping can be as primitive as spending the night in a small tent or a spacious RV. Then there's painting and Zen drawing. I tried the latter for a while and found it very rewarding. It requires absolutely no talent because the purpose is not to produce a work of art, but to get you to see things you normally wouldn't notice. It doesn't have to be done in nature, but that was my favorite environment to practice in. It works as a great stress reducer indoors, too, but the effect is magnified several times outdoors.

There are great nature videos and CDs available, and several TV channels have some fine shows, too. Yes, I know it's TV. If well done, they can be great stress relievers. However, if you have ever looked into the Grand Canyon, after seeing it in pictures or videos a thousand times before, you realize there is no substitute for the real thing.

Planning ahead for the unexpected

This stress-reducing technique covers a lot of territory, from having good health insurance to leaving an umbrella in the car in case it rains.

When I was writing this chapter, I moved my computer from the office to the kitchen counter to clean off my desk. I like to work at the kitchen counter from time to time. I neglected to take my back up device, too, even though it is only about the size of a wallet. Three days later, I went out for breakfast and returned to find the computer off because of a brief electrical power blackout. When I double clicked to the Stress Chapter, the pages were blank. I tried another chapter I had been working on, and it was also blank. I took a deep breath and told myself, "OK, I'm going to lose this week's work, but everything else was backed up." I was a little put out, but not really stressed. Imagine though, if I hadn't had the backup device! So I decided to restart the computer, and like magic, everything was back to normal. I retrieved the backup device, plugged it in and got back to work. All was well with the universe!

Of course we can't plan for everything; and we really shouldn't, as I often remind my wife. Actually, Colette loves my spontaneity. The hurricane victim that had no flood insurance saved a few hundred dollars each year. However, when the 100-year flood comes early, the different stress levels on him and that of his insured neighbor are quite dramatic.

The Crohn's patient that enjoys the pleasure of spicy chicken wings, French fries and ice cream just before bed has a stress level on their face dramatically different from that of the Crohnie that thought ahead and had baked chicken breast, baked potato and spinach salad 3 or 4 hours before retiring for the night. I know, I have seen both faces in my mirror. The first is not pretty.

One of our favorite trips and purchases took place with almost no planning. One evening, sitting at my computer on a Trailer Sailor forum, someone mentioned there was a good buy on a sailboat in Idaho. I inquired and received pictures and description via email. I woke at 5 a.m. and replied that I wanted to buy the boat. When I called to confirm later that morning, there were already three other offers on the waiting list. Because of the chance of October snows in the Rockies, we started our road trip 2 days later. We not only had a fun adventure and met some great people, we bought a beautiful boat. The die-hard planners never had a chance.

A wise person knows when to plan for the future and when to be in the present. A healthy life has both.

Going with the flow

A corollary to "being prepared," is dealing with troubling situations beyond our control in a positive way. When managing Crohn's disease, you have to accept that there is an ebb and flow to life. Being a sailor, I have some awareness of the impact of tides, and know when it makes sense to go against the flow and when it is better to wait for the currents to change.

Being diagnosed with Crohn's disease and deciding to change nothing in one's life except taking medication is, in my opinion, going against the flow. It may work for a while, but at some point you have to pay the piper.

The year I had three intestinal blockages and three hospital stays, I went against the flow. Abdominal pain barely slowed me. A grimace, a hand on my offending cells, and I marched on. John Wayne would have been proud.

Eventually, I learned to go with the flow. I paired my business down to where I had fewer employees and I chose my clients more carefully. Revenue decreased, but so did my stress. Interestingly, profits went up, another stress reducer. Of course, there were always times when the flow or something was not in my favor, so I used other stress management tools to get me through those periods.

Meditation, breathing, yoga and other exercise

I have discussed yoga and Crohn's at length, but there are other Eastern practices, such as "soft" martial arts, which can provide similar benefits for improving health and reducing stress. Two that are increasing in popularity in the United States are tai chi and qigong.

Tai Chi is a rhythmic pattern of movements that are coordinated with breathing to help one achieve a sense of inner calm. It is a combination of movement for fluidity, meditation and martial arts. Today there are many styles, and it can be very beautiful to watch. The most obvious differences between tai chi and yoga are more movement in the former and more work sitting and lying on the floor in the latter.

Qigong involves dynamic training, static training, meditative training, and the use of external agents (tai chi is actually a subsidiary practice of qigong). The dynamic training involves carefully choreographed fluid movement coordinated with the breath. The static training resembles yoga because postures are held for some time. The meditative training focuses on the breath, visualization, mantra and philosophical concepts. The use of external agents by many Qigong practitioners may mean ingestion of herbs, and massage.

Summary

According to Hans Selye, "It's not stress that kills us, it is our reaction to it." Or, as the Mayo Clinic's website suggests, stress may not cause Crohn's, but it can trigger flare-ups and make symptoms worse. It recommends physical exercise, biofeedback, as well as relaxation and breath exercises, yoga, and meditation to manage that stress. I couldn't agree more.

Chapter 10
REST, ENERGY AND SLEEP

A good laugh and a long sleep are the two best cures for anything.
—Irish Proverb

One thing I have discovered in my journey with Crohn's is the importance of rest and sleep. When I was younger, working 60 or more hours a week and raising a family, it was often difficult to get sleep because I had too much on my mind. Besides, if you are a Type A person, like me, you may look on sleep as one of the obstacles to overcome in order to reach your goals. However, if you are a really smart Type A person, who has undergone some self-reflection, you may realize that sleep is actually an ally.

There are some people who require less than normal sleep. Peter the Great, the 18th century Russian czar, needed only 5 hours a night. With extra time on his hands, he thought a great deal about his country, instituted massive changes, modernizing Russia, and brought it closer to Western European standards of the time.

But for the most part, there is no need to envy people who have energy to spare and seem to require little sleep. Usually they are loaded up on coffee, sodas and sugar or operate on emotional energy producers like fear or anger. When I was in graduate school, I was working three jobs while taking a full-time load of courses. I'd wait until the last moment possible to get really focused on papers and other assignments. I would tell myself I had enough time to get them done and would do it by engaging my adrenals. It worked great, and I made mostly A's. Of course, I was also diagnosed with Crohn's about the time I completed my master's degree. To what degree my way of working played a role in that, I will never know. There may be many reasons why I developed Crohn's. However, I am sure that chronic stress, whether self-inflicted or created by others, is not good for the immune system. Pushing one's self too far on a regular basis may not be wise for a healthy individual, and it is especially risky for someone with an inflammatory bowel disorder.

It may be that Crohn's disease, as an autoimmune disorder, makes people more tired because their bodies produce too much inflammation. Medical science has demonstrated, and it is common sense, that when our bodies produce chemicals to fight infection, one of the side effects is increased fatigue. This forces us to conserve energy in order to help us recover. Think of it as one of the mechanisms developed by evolution to protect us from ourselves. Imagine if we had a serious infection and normal, or more than normal, energy. We would be working or playing harder than ever, and our bodies would be using up their resources to support the muscles instead of concentrating them on the infection in order to heal it. So we're fortunate that our bodies function in ways that allow us to survive rather than glow brightly and burn out.

It has been confirmed by medical studies that sleep helps the cardiovascular system, contributes to the regulation of blood sugar, boosts the immune system, and aids the skin—the body's largest organ. Nighttime, when most of us rest, is also when the parasympathetic system takes over. Remember our sympathetic system, which we use to varying degrees thoughout the waking hours, is associated with expending energy and tearing down the body. The parasympathetic system, which rules as we sleep, works to nurture the body and regenerate body tissue. It also allows the digestive system to operate at its peak performance levels.

In addition, some of the best mental processing occurs while sleeping. As a child, I was pretty good at math, but sometimes I would not be able to solve a problem. If I went to bed, often the following morning I would wake up with the solution. The same is true today when I face a difficult problem or decision. If I sleep on it, I often wake up the next morning with a clear understanding of what needs to be done.

Getting Plenty of Rest

Like Thomas Alva Edison, the great American inventor who gave us the phonograph, the incandescent light bulb, and the movie camera among many others, I am a great believer in taking naps. When working intensely on one of his inventions, Edison would curl up for 10 minutes at a time on or beneath his work desk, wake up refreshed, and tackle the problem anew.

I have found that if I allow myself a nap in the afternoon—but no more than 20 minutes—I can overcome the fatigue that creeps up at that time of day. It beats getting wired on coffee or other stimulants.

When I feel fatigued, it is not always possible to tell if it is because of Crohn's or for another reason. It doesn't really matter. How you deal with it should be the same. If it is because of overwork and I push on, chances are the stress associated with that will negatively impact my Crohn's. There are times I may not have much choice. If I am getting ready for a big event at work or out on the water, I will keep going. Sometimes I do fine, yet other times, I pay a price afterward. However, if my work schedule is flexible, I take time off or slow down my efforts. If I am working out at the gym, I focus on less difficult exercise or stretching, or I go home. The important thing is to be smart about our choices.

But nothing beats a good night's sleep.

Here are some ways to help you get to do that. First, allocate enough time for sleep. Eight to nine hours is what most people need. If you have to be up at 5 a.m. to get ready for work, that means going to bed no later than 9 p.m. Make sure you eat your evening meal early and keep it light. Avoid dense, not easily digested foods. The top ten foods hardest to digest are ice cream, citrus drinks, mashed potatoes (because of the cream or milk), spicy foods, beans, chocolate, onions, fried foods, broccoli and cabbage and sugar free gum. This is especially important for people with Crohn's. If you have a sweet tooth, indulge at lunch, not at dinner.

On the weekends, Colette and I usually eat later and more and often than not, have a dessert. As a result, I almost never sleep as well on the weekends as during the week.

Stay away from anything that will stimulate the nervous system near bedtime. Avoid coffee, tea, arguments, and vigorous mental or physical activities. The full brightness light setting on the screen of any self-luminous tablet, cell phone or computer may affect your melatonin levels and, therefore, your sleep. Simply set the brightness level at about half or less intensity.

A gentle walk or a light read is great just before bed. If it is something that is going to get you going, like a good suspense novel or action packed movie on TV, put it aside or record it for earlier the next day.

Make sure your bedroom is quiet and dark. I like the "white" noise of a small fan to muffle outside sounds. Have the right temperature set for your body. If your spouse has a hot metabolism and yours is colder by nature, try warmer pajamas and direct a fan on the other side of the bed. Pick out the right mattress and pillows. If your box springs squeak, replace them. If the budget is a problem, put a sheet of plywood between the springs and mattress. If that does not work, maybe the plywood can be put directly on the bed slats and the mattress on top of that. Just make sure your bedroom and bed are the best they can be for rest and sleep.

❦ *Chapter 11*
RELATIONSHIPS

One of the biggest challenges with Crohn's is relationships. You may appear completely normal to most people, but if you act like everyone else to fit in and belong, it will make your life miserable. If you protect yourself, you'll stand out as different, and some people have a hard time dealing with that. In my experience, it becomes less difficult with age, but it never goes away completely.

Even close friends often don't get it. The more normal you appear, the less they seem to understand it. After 50, so many people are on medication, they often ask why I just don't take more pills. There is increasing awareness now that medicating isn't always the best approach to health, but most of the people I've met don't seem to realize that drugs just treat the symptoms. They haven't come around to the point of view that it is to our advantage to reduce the need for those pills by our actions. Believe me, if I thought taking pills would solve the problem, I'd be the first in line at the pharmacy.

Marriage and Significant Others

Obviously, everything I have been describing gets magnified a hundred fold in an intimate relationship.

Since I have been married three times, I have a variety of experiences to draw on in this regard. Spouse number one was before Crohn's.

I had known her in 7th grade and started to date her in college. Our marriage did not survive my being a young lieutenant in Vietnam.

Spouse number two was blind-sided by my Crohn's diagnosis. She had met and fallen in love with this healthy, hard working, and hard playing guy, but after barely a year together, I became very sick, and we went through many ups and downs together as we both learned what it meant to live with a chronic illness. She may have felt somewhat cheated, and I don't blame her for that. It was hard for her because she just wanted to be normal and have a normal husband. We were married a little more than 15 years, and all but the last two were very good.

Five years later, I met my lovely Colette. I told her about my Crohn's disease early on in our relationship. Having had to deal with her own health challenges, she was very empathetic. Her story is interesting and inspiring. Just out of college, 22 years old, and suffering from allergies, mood swings, irregular periods, and weight loss, she saw an endocrinologist, a specialist who treats hormone imbalances.

A CAT scan and blood test revealed a grapefruit sized ovarian cyst and led to a diagnosis of severe red meat allergy. An OB/GYN exam showed pre-cancerous cervical cells. The endocrinologist prescribed pharmaceuticals to suppress and control the ovarian cyst and strongly suggested that red meat be stricken from her diet. The gynecologist advised surgery to remove the pre-cancerous cells.

A friend recommended that Colette see a licensed naturopathic doctor (ND) who might have a different approach. According to the American Association of Naturopathic Physicians, NDs take all of the same basic science courses as MDs, but also study holistic approaches, disease prevention, nutrition, homeopathic medicine, botanical medicine, psychology and counseling. They take professional board exams and are licensed by a state or jurisdiction as primary care, general practice physicians.

The ND prescribed an organic vegetarian diet consisting of fruits, vegetables, whole grains, beans and other legumes. In addition, Colette was to exercise, meditate, read about health, and stand in front of a mirror every day to get to know her body and see how it was changing. After several discussions with her MDs, Colette decided to postpone the surgery and not take the prescription drugs for a trial period.

The program not only cured her allergies, mood swings, irregular periods and weight loss, a gynecological exam six weeks later found no pre-cancerous cells. Follow up CAT scans showed no evidence of the ovarian cyst. Sometimes angels cross our paths. Colette's was a naturopathic doctor, and mine was Colette.

After the Nirvana stage, and our romance settled into a more tranquil relationship, Colette wanted to help me with my diet. She understood that you can't deal with a chronic health issue without modifying your behavior. Since my Crohn's diagnosis, I had come a long way in my health awareness concerning diet and health, but she took me to a higher level. She also found *Eating Right for a Bad Gut*, the book that has helped me the most to deal with Crohn's disease, and she read it first! I could not ask for anyone better as far as understanding and support.

However, even Colette sometimes doesn't get what it is that I need. Although we agree on most of what we eat, it took her several years to accept that certain high fiber foods were bad for me and that the peels of just about everything—including potatoes, apples and tomatoes—gave me problems.

In addition, virtually all raw vegetables work for her; mine must be cooked more thoroughly. Coarse whole wheat agrees with her, I need finely ground whole wheat. We triple rinse our beans because of me. She likes unpasteurized cheese; I like pasteurized everything. Basically, I baby my digestive system; she treats hers like the champion gut it is.

I have found that it is best to be patient and gently communicate my needs. It is important to accept that the person living with someone with Crohn's often has to accept things that seem counterintuitive so they probably won't always get it the first or second time. Someday your spouse will mostly get it. If not, you'll just have to be that much more determined and perhaps learn how to cook for yourself.

Ultimately, the greatest gift a spouse can provide is not helping with the right foods, but being understanding of your situation. If your spouse looks at you with scorn or ridicules what you eat, even the best food won't digest well.

Friends

Close friends are like husbands and wives. They will accept you as you are and need to be. If they can't do that, they can't be close friends anymore. Chances are, though, they won't be a problem, especially if you see them fairly often. Remember, they don't "get it" the way you do, so work with them. Be patient, explain and educate. If they aren't willing to work with you, then they probably aren't a healthy choice of friends (psychologically as well as physically), and it may be time to move on. Now, if your spouse or significant other is more concerned about hurting the friend's feelings than your health, and the two of you can't work it out, it might be time for some counseling.

Casual friends and acquaintances can be more of a problem; they may have a harder time understanding your issues. But because you both have less invested in the relationship, it usually can be worked out over time fairly easily. Still, you will need to be forever on guard.

My wife and I attended a gathering recently, where the "chef" was a bit put out when I politely turned down the barbecued ribs and corn and asked me, "Can you eat anything?" I smiled and moved on, not bothering to comment. However, at other shindigs my sharing that I have Crohn's has led to warm, interesting, and rewarding conversations.

Just remember, there are sensitive and insensitive people out there. Most want to be empathetic and responsive. Once in a while, I meet someone, however, who makes such boorish remarks that I ignore them or occasionally return the "favor" with a mocking comment of my own.

If you don't have a flair for sarcasm, don't worry; it is probably to your advantage in the bigger scheme of things. Sarcasm can take over your personality, if you're not careful.

Be wary of people who are energy leeches. These are the folks that create a negative, chaotic atmosphere. They can push your buttons and feed off your energy by upsetting you—it energizes them. Years ago, I heard an interview with Norman Mailer, an American author who had an Ernest Hemingway-type personality. He loved to fight, drink and carouse. He engaged in verbal jousting even more than the occasional drunken brawl. At some point, the journalist asked him if his lifestyle was harmful to his health. Although Mailer was often a difficult person, he was also a thoughtful man. He replied that he imagined those who lived with him, and people like him, were more at risk healthwise, and he believed he may have been the reason his wife got cancer.

Dating and Social Life

Despite a host of websites and social media networks to facilitate meeting that special other person, hooking up with others is more than just a virtual experience. If you are single and looking for a partner or future spouse, going out for dinner or a movie is an essential part of the getting-to-know-you dance. This can present a major quandary for someone with Crohn's. Say you are on a date and there is something you know you shouldn't eat, like popcorn at the movies, do you say, "I don't like popcorn," or "I am not hungry," or do you spill the beans regarding the real reason?

In the beginning, I believe a compromise is the best strategy. You don't have to go into detail. You can say, "I don't digest popcorn well" Or "I have a challenged digestive system and popcorn is one of the things I have to stay away from." If there is something you can eat at the movies and you get that instead, you don't even have to deal with the issue.

More importantly, as the relationship develops, when and how do you "let the cat out of the bag" about your Crohn's? My philosophy is there is no reason to bring it up first thing, but waiting too long isn't a good idea either. After all, good relationships are built on a foundation of honesty. Having a plan for when the time is right makes good sense. There is a risk of rejection, of course, which is why so many people postpone talking about it, but that's not a good reason to keep it a secret for too long. Give it your best shot and tell your new friend about your chronic illness. If that scares him or her away, you are better off knowing it early on, even if it means having to spend some time alone. Be thankful and move on.

Family

We were planning a family vacation with my wife's brother and two sisters and their families. Everyone liked camping, except one sister, so we opted for a long weekend get-together at a campground, while she and her family rented a deluxe cabin. The rest of us had nice tents and camping gear, so we all expected to have a great time. One of the sisters suggested we share all meals and rotate who prepares them. If we had gone along with that, then I would have been either sick or hungry for the entire family vacation. If it had been only one meal, I could have eaten something beforehand, and nibbled on what I could tolerate at the meal, but this was a long weekend!

We wanted to fit in and enjoy our time with the group. Our solution was to remind our relatives that I have Crohn's disease, so Colette and I would prepare our own breakfasts and lunches, and either bring them to the gatherings, or eat first, and come with a cup of coffee. For dinners, we would bring our own main dish and a side to share. The others could combine their efforts, and we would all eat together.

The key to making it work is having a spouse who is both understanding and practical, being tactful and honest with the others, and having reasonable family members who can be flexible.

How to Deal with Relationship Conflicts

I have heard many times that it takes two people to destroy a marriage or relationship. I disagree. I believe it takes two people to *have* a good marriage or good relationship. One person will have to take the first step and give more, but the other person has to give some as well.

One issue my wife and I had to deal with was that she liked to eat her main meal late, and I wanted and needed to eat it early. Eventually, we worked out a solution. During the week, we simply fix and eat our evening meal separately. Friday, Saturday and Sunday evenings, we do it together, both of us compromising on the time. I suppose another option would be to keep to the same, separate schedule the whole week, but we both value eating together enough to make the necessary adjustments part of the time.

The most important thing in such negotiations is to communicate one's needs. The next most important thing is to listen to the other person's needs. After that, both parties must compromise where they can and then live up to their obligations. Of course, this is easier said than done and requires work and a mutual generosity of spirit.

Here is how Colette and I worked out one of our food differences. While she likes most vegetables barely cooked and I want mine well done, cooking everything in two pots is not an ideal solution. So after a few years (nobody said it was fast and easy), we started cutting veggies like broccoli and cauliflower into very small pieces for me and into big chunks for her. The smaller sized vegetables cook more quickly and thoroughly. For greens such as chard, we start steaming mine and put hers in later. It is not difficult to keep them separate in the pot. In both examples, mine are more cooked and thus easier for me to digest.

Counseling

If all else fails, seeking professional advice may be required. I have gone to counselors twice. The first time was for two sessions prior to my first divorce. They were very helpful and eye opening. The second time was before my second divorce. Again, the sessions were beneficial. Maybe marriage counselors should be called divorce counselors. In my experience, they can help in the process of separation and often make it more amiable.

Another experience I had with a counselor was more informal and less positive. It happened at a dinner my wife and I had with a psychologist and her husband. Discussion turned to a relative of hers, whom Colette and I had met previously. She had been divorced for some time, had been raising two very nice and smart teenage sons on her own, and was dating a man who was causing her a great deal of heartache. He was controlling and self-absorbed, and barely tolerated the boys. The psychologist said she thought the two should get married; that a bad marriage would be better for her relative than breaking up because that would be a blow to her self esteem. She kept defending her position over vehement disagreement by the rest of us. I, certainly, would never consider going to her for counsel, nor would I recommend anyone else to do so.

My point is—be careful. There are some great, thoroughly-professional counselors out there, but many who have their own issues and may not be suited to you. Don't assume every counselor will work for you. Research first, then go for a tryout, until you find the right one. Trust your gut on this—if you're meeting with someone that seems odd and rubs you the wrong way, it's probably not a good fit. Get away as quickly as possible and keep looking.

Expectations and Sense of Humor

I find I get the most frustrated when my expectations are high and my sense of humor is low. For example, we attended our annual weekend event with our online Trailer Sailor club at Cedar Key, Florida. Usually, we are on our respective boats, but at this event, most of us stay at various hotels or condos. There are planned get-togethers and meals on Friday and Saturday nights. Most years, we have not been able to eat the main dish, which was Polish sausage.

On this occasion, the Friday night offering was pulled pork sandwiches provided by one of our members at a community center. We ate dinner first and went over later to socialize. It was fun to see our friends.

The Saturday night outdoor get-together is the big event of the weekend, and for the first time, the planned menu was to our liking. Instead of the usual grilled sausages, the caterers were offering a great seafood meal. My taste buds were all set for grilled shrimp and other marine delights.

Imagine then, how I felt when we found out that the main entrée was pulled pork, and that the shrimp dish was swimming with Polish sausage. I literally dropped my glass of wine. It turned out that the original caterer had suddenly gone out of business. The last minute change of menu for the event had been announced on the club's forum, but I had missed the notice.

Fortunately, with some dinner rolls, dessert and wine, not to mention Colette's ability to accept such glitches with equanimity, my sense of humor eventually kicked in, helping me to overcome my disappointment and allowing us to have a great evening. I now refer to it as the "pulled-pork gathering" when in the company of close friends.

So regarding family, friends, other relationships, and food, keeping expectations low is the best strategy. A simple, but effective, tactic is to eat a little before going to an event or someone's house. It is a lot easier to watch others enjoying a good meal if the stomach is not empty. After that, improvise, and if all else fails, laugh.

❧ *Chapter 12*
CAREERS

Having a chronic health problem makes careers and work life considerably more challenging. Someone with Crohn's disease may want to think twice before pursuing the 10 most stressful jobs of 2013 as published on *www.careercast.com*:

- Enlisted soldier
- Military general
- Firefighter
- Commercial airline pilot
- Public relations executive
- Senior corporate executive
- Photojournalist
- Newspaper reporter
- Taxi driver
- Police officer

However, three-time Olympic sprint kayaker Carrie Johnson and General Dwight D. Eisenhower didn't let Crohn's get in the way of their careers. I believe we Crohnies can pursue just about any profession or occupation we pick.

My Career Choices

I wanted a career that was creative, took place outside, had lots of variety, challenged me, and would allow me to earn enough money to live well. It took me several trials, both successful and not so successful, to find one that I loved.

I was diagnosed with Crohn's about the time I completed my MBA. By then I had built a successful janitorial service to pay the bills, but I didn't like it all that much. I was trying to figure out what to do when a Western Auto franchise became available for sale. I had worked there part time during my undergraduate college days and knew the business. Although my confidence was a bit fragile because of the recent diagnosis, I decided to see if I could swing a loan and become a merchant. With my background, education and business plan, I bought a $100,000 franchise with $5,000 and a signature. I was a respected businessman in Murfreesboro, Tennessee. The Western Auto was a store that sold a combination of hardware, auto parts, appliances, tires, bicycles and toys. The profit margins were slim, the rent was high, and the only way to make it work was on the finance charges of the items sold on credit.

To make a long story short, it was the worst possible time to get into that business. The economy went south. Many people who had accounts at the auto store for 20 or more years lost their jobs. The economy took its toll on marriages, too, and long-time store accounts often went unpaid. A Walmart opened up a few blocks away—the kiss of death for many small businesses. Interest rates on commercial loans went from 6% to 20%. Two and a half years later, I was broke, in debt big time, and once again, trying to decide what to do.

One of my former employees who had become a good friend said he would help me start a commercial lawn mowing business. He would be the mechanic and part time worker. I started calling manufacturing plants and large apartment complexes to drum up business. To my surprise, it only took 2 months before I had a successful company going. And here was the kicker. You'd think that being a commercial lawn maintenance company owner, manager and operator would be much harder work than being a merchant. But in truth, for me it was easier and much more profitable. There were times I worked too hard and paid the price, but overall, it was less stressful.

I went on to take courses in landscaping design, turf management, and landscaping plants. Over the years, I created beautiful environments, solved irrigation system problems, managed people, and worked outside much of the time. I kept growing my business and for the most part, loved it.

I learned two huge valuable lessons in regard to Crohn's disease and careers. The first—don't make a big career move right after learning that you have a chronic disease. The second—it is important to have a career you love, even if the work seems harder because the stress of toiling hour after hour, day after day, year after year at something you don't like is the hardest work of all.

For me, being self-employed became one of the tools for managing Crohn's. Not everyone is suited to being an entrepreneur, but if you have the skill set, including the right personality for it, I highly recommend it.

As with everything in life, there are pros and cons. One downside is long hours, especially in the first 5 to 10 years. On the other hand, you have flexibility in scheduling your work time. On a day when you feel bad or suffer a period of fatigue, you can work for 1 or 2 hours. If you are feeling great, put in 12 hours if you want to. The only time you have to eat out is when you are taking a client to lunch. If you pay, you can almost always choose the restaurant. Similarly, if a vendor treats you, you can often choose the eating establishment. The better you train your employees, the more freedom you have.

In the early days because I worked long hours, I often ate fast food. My doctor, in his ignorance, supported it, and that was a big mistake. The double cheeseburger with bacon and fries on the side was the meal

I ate before my first trip to the emergency room, followed by several days in the hospital. Years later and not long after my first surgery, I began to improve my diet. Limiting my fast food intake was a big key to not having a second surgery.

I also found out the hard way that taking late night phone calls is not a healthy thing. Since I ran my landscape business out of my home, any signal that I had a phone call was like a fire alarm. I had to either answer it or check the message because I would imagine the worst possible news, either at that time or worse yet, at two in the morning. If a client left a message to call, I worried about losing that contract even though 99 times out of 100 my worries were completely unfounded.

Eventually, I never took calls after 8 p.m., sometimes even earlier, and it had no negative effect on my relationships, friends, business, or family whatsoever. I had to make sure not to check my phone "after hours," which took some reprogramming. I also turned off any signals that would alert me that I got a message, like special sounds on mobile phones.

You may feel that there are one or more people that must be able to reach you at any time—perhaps the nurse of an ailing parent or your kids. For those cases, I suggest getting a separate unlisted phone number for them to call.

If you are the type of person that can't stand not immediately picking up every phone call you get, or if you have to be a part of everything and can't adjust, then this part of my approach to managing Crohn's is going to be especially difficult for you. It took me considerable time to fix this one, too. I had to learn to control my need to be on top of everything right away. I did this largely through techniques I learned in yoga and self-help books.

Being Employed

Crohn's and the workplace can be tricky. The main issue is whether or not to inform your boss and teammates that you have a chronic illness and risk termination. Although it may or may not be illegal to fire someone because they have Crohn's, the hassles of suing, if it happens, may not be worth the aggravation to your health.

If you are in the probationary period of a new job and wish to keep your illness secret, you may have to use stealth tactics. The most challenging times are lunches out or meetings where the meal is catered. The issues are similar to socializing with friends and relatives. If there is nothing you can eat without less than desirable consequences, you have several options. A bad one, in my opinion, is to eat what everyone else does and risk getting sick. Another is to eat a little and maybe get a little sick. A third is to order what others are having and just push it around your plate. That usually works pretty well. Or you might say you will just have a glass of tea or whatever.

At some point, you probably will have to spill the beans about your Crohn's. Once you are a valued member of the team, it usually won't matter.

There are lots of places that accept people with health challenges, from government offices, to non-profit agencies. Anything you're uniquely good at will be a passport to special allowances. If you can sell cars, nothing else matters. In fact, sales may be the most equal opportunity career there is. The same is true if you are a talented research scientist or musician. However, if you are an average Joe or Jane in the workplace, you may have to pick a job that accepts limitations or learn techniques to camouflage them. Time and good performance will reduce your need to cover up your diet and health challenges.

If the job is not really the right fit for you and you are just hanging in there until the position of your dreams comes along, it gets trickier. You will experience considerable stress, aggravated by the fact that you probably feel unhappy about your circumstances. My recommendation is to get out as quickly as you can. It may be scary initially, but in my experience—and that of others I have watched go through it—it is better to leave an uncomfortable nest sooner rather than later. One of the things that's great about our country, still, is that there are many opportunities you can pursue. And most people have greater options than they initially believe they have.

Anytime I am feeling sorry for myself regarding Crohn's disease, I think of Stephen Hawking, the English theoretical physicist and cosmologist who has a motor neuron disease that has almost completely paralyzed him and requires him to communicate through a speech-generating device. Yet, he has done significant scientific work, written popular books, married twice, and has three children.

I also think of one of my wife's friends who acquired lupus at a relatively young age and later, cancer. She continues to amaze my wife and me as she maintains a positive attitude, strives to improve her skills and advances in her chosen career. She recently earned her Ph.D., works as an arbitrator for a university and loves singing with a women's choir.

The U.S. Army has a great slogan in its commercials: "Be All You Can Be." Most of us achieve only a fraction of what we're capable. While Crohn's disease is an obstacle, it doesn't have to prevent us from following our dreams.

❧ Chapter 13
WORKING WITH HEALTH PROVIDERS

Working with people in the medical profession is similar to working with any service provider. You are the consumer and they are the suppliers. The difference is that, because of their expertise, physicians and institutions like hospitals have more power in the equation. Although most are compassionate, intelligent, and dedicated to their profession, on many occasions, ego, callousness, and/or bureaucratic inefficiency can get in the way. What that means to patients is that they must be especially vigilant in making sure to get the best service possible.

When I lived in Murfreesboro, a small city of about 100,000, I personally knew many of the doctors. When I moved to Southwest Florida, I knew none and didn't have friends or other local contacts to get a recommendation for a good general practitioner. I went on the Internet and picked one. It wasn't the right choice, so I picked another, and he worked out great. When I went looking for a gastroenterologist, the first one I found was arrogant and unreliable. I soon chose another, and have been very pleased with him. Unlike the first candidate, he not only took 30 minutes on my first visit, he actually listened to what I had to say.

The Health Care Pyramid

There are many types of health providers. Medical doctors (MDs) are at the top of the pyramid. Doctors of Osteopathy (ODs) are near the top, and in a few locales, at the top. ODs get additional training in manipulating the body for certain health benefits. Among the MDs and ODs, the specialists have more prestige and usually earn more. Just below the MDs are the physician assistants (PAs) and nurse practitioners (NPs), then the nurses (RNs). Nurses, in my opinion, are both the backbone and the soul of the medical community.

That is the conventional medical community hierarchy.

Alternative health providers practice outside the domain of the conventional medical community. I have gone to acupuncturists and chiropractors. Just as in the conventional medical community, I have received poor, good, and excellent service, so I am very selective about whom I visit.

Acupuncturists, especially, have been a great help to me, both in California and in Tennessee. On my first visit, I could actually feel energy pulsating through the damaged area of my small intestine. During subsequent treatments, I usually felt nothing except a sense of calm. More importantly, after my visits, I felt more energy and less discomfort. In the past decade, acupuncture has become more recognized by the American medical establishment, and it is being taught at some medical schools. If it were covered by my insurance, I would use it more often.

Important Physician Qualities

In my opinion, having someone who listens is one of the most important qualities in a physician. If your doctor is good, she or he will be busy. That doesn't justify not taking the time to really listen. Would you go to a barber or hair stylist that didn't listen to your request? When I grew up in the 50's and 60's, that was the practice with boys' haircuts in my hometown. No matter what the barber was told, everybody got white sidewalls. One of my friends even took a picture of what he wanted to the barber and got the same haircut as everyone else.

A doctor who doesn't listen won't realize that you want to be involved in your health, but if you have a chronic disease like Crohn's, it is essential that you become a partner in your health care.

So "Buyer Beware" is the motto I go by. When I go to any health care provider, I try to get as much of the following questions answered ahead of time via the Internet, or directly from them before I get on their table for an examination.

My questions include:

- What, where, when and how much training have you had?
- What license do you have, and what was required to get it?
- What, where, when and how much of your training was working directly with patients or was it observing them being helped by other physicians?
- What, where, and how long have you been practicing?
- How many Crohn's patients have you seen, and what kind of success have you had with them?
- What treatments do you use with Crohn's patients, and how often do you recommend they have a treatment?

My experience is that the good and well trained health providers love to answer these questions, and the ones that have a problem with them are not worth a second visit.

I suggest reading a book like *The Not So Patient Advocate* by Ellen Menard, which provides extensive examples of how to talk to your health care providers—from GPs to physicians in the emergency room—in order to develop a team approach to your medical care. Among her many suggestions, she counsels bringing a written list of questions because many of us draw a blank at a time when we feel concerned about our well being.

Then there is the money issue. Health care in this country is big business, and unless you have the wherewithal to afford supplemental insurance, it will behoove you to check the costs before you have anything more than routine care done.

For example, it is a lot more expensive to have an out-patient procedure performed at a hospital than an approved clinic that is not connected to the hospital. In most cases, treatment is just as good at one as the other. Recently, my wife was having some pain, and it was eventually decided she needed an MRI. The doctor's office scheduled the procedure at a clinic. When Colette called the insurance company to make sure this clinic was on the approved list, she was told the procedure would cost $300 because it was affiliated with a hospital. After some research, she discovered a radiology clinic 5 minutes from our home, where the cost would be $200. After checking with the doctor's office, she was able to schedule the MRI at the more convenient and less expensive location. Doing her homework saved us $100. Our lesson, always call the insurance company before getting a procedure.

Since World War II, health care has evolved dramatically. In fact, health care has evolved dramatically in the past 20 years. Advancing medical technology may be offset by poorer diets. Doctors may be better trained than ever, but there may be less availability, especially in certain areas or specialties. Health care laws may open up more medical services to some, but make health care more expensive for others. Computers and communication advances allow for telemedicine but will regulators and special interests allow it to be used? Two things we can be sure about our medical care systems are that they will constantly change, and some of the changes will be good and some bad.

Mahatma Gandhi said, "Nobody can hurt me without my permission." I doubt my will is as strong as Gandhi's, but with the challenges he faced, he believed that attitude surely can go a long way in keeping a few bad health "professionals" from hurting us, and opening up the space in our lives for some great health care providers to come our way.

🌿 *Chapter 14*
CONCLUSION

If you are new to Crohn's and haven't had to think much about how to deal with a chronic illness, it is likely that you may feel overwhelmed by all the information. It took me years to develop a way of living and dealing with the disease, that worked for me. Much of it I discovered by trial and error. In other instances, I had to overcome old-fashioned, but authoritatively-presented views.

It doesn't have to be that painstaking of a process for you.

Let's imagine we are getting ready for a wonderful trip, a fantastic voyage. We have a burden to carry, but we really want to reach our destination. The destination, our destiny, is to live a great life with or without Crohn's disease. Taking it one step at a time, and not necessarily in this order, I recommend doing the following:

- Recognize what Crohn's is, not making it better or worse than it is.

- Understand the importance of a positive attitude, and either nurture the one you have, or begin to develop the one you need.

- Look at your diet and focus on developing one that is not destructive, but enjoyable, and supports your short and long term health goals.

- Develop a weeklong meal plan. Be specific.

- Decide what your exercise goals and methods are.

- Make a weekly plan of what, when, where, why, and how to exercise. Update and modify as needed.

- Buy a book or DVD on yoga or attend a class, using what you learned in the yoga chapter to guide that process. If yoga is not for you, learn other relaxation, breath, biofeedback, and stretching techniques.

- Meditate 15 to 30 minutes a day, 5 to 7 days a week.

- Use one or more stress management tools that work for you. Add a new tool every week until you have an effective stress-buster tool box.

- Set aside time every day to take a nap or rest in a way that you desire.

- Look at your relationships and evaluate which ones help you and which ones are destructive. Find a way to get the strength to improve or eliminate the destructive ones.

- Look at your career and either appreciate it, or begin making short and long term plans to change it.

- Evaluate your health care providers and change them if you are not happy with them.

- Be realistic and realize there will be setbacks. When you trip over a root or become winded because the grade is too steep, stop, evaluate your route, and your pace. When rested or healed, smile, appreciate the beauty of the scenery along the way, and realize Crohn's disease is just one of the burdens we carry. Then take one more step toward the destination you have chosen.

I have organized this book in the order I consider the most useful way to proceed, but feel free to create your own route for your health journey.

There are no easy answers, but living with Crohn's doesn't have to be a difficult, traumatic process.

Remember, a person with one health problem is usually healthier than a person with no health problem.

MAY YOU LIVE WELL!

❧ ACKNOWLEDGMENTS

I would like to thank my wife, Colette, who believed I would, could and should write this book. When I wavered, she never did. Also, I deeply appreciate her assistance with the copy editing and proofing of this book. Her attention to detail is outstanding!

I would like to thank my editor and producer, Chris Angermann, who saw the value of this book. He guided and assisted in the refining and polishing way beyond the call of duty. His patience, diligence and quest for excellence is much appreciated. His oversight, putting everything together and seeing the book through to publication, has been invaluable.

Thanks to all the great health care providers—the doctors, the nurses, and the acupuncturists for their dedication, years of training, and compassion. A special thanks goes to the hospital nurses for their empathy and care.

Thanks to my yoga teachers who taught me to how to be engaged and relaxed at the same time, and how to breathe.

Thanks to my yoga students whose confidence in me made me want to be the best teacher I could be.

And finally, thanks to my family and friends who choose not to see me as a man with Crohn's disease, but as a man who lives mindfully, with an entrepreneurial spirit, a sense of humor, and a love for adventure.

For more information
and links to further resources,
go to

www.theartoflivingwell.com.

www.ingramcontent.com/pod-product-compliance
Lightning Source LLC
Chambersburg PA
CBHW021010090426
42738CB00007B/739